# The Art of the Brazilian Butt Lift

Mark Youssef, MD

Foreword by Dr. Miami,
aka Michael Salzhauer, MD

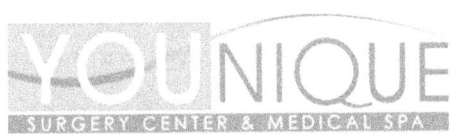

The Art of the Brazilian Butt Lift

Copyright © 2019 by Mark Youssef, MD

All rights reserved. No portion of this book may be reproduced in any form without permission from the publisher, except as permitted by U.S. copyright law. For more information, go to:

https://www.youniquecosmeticsurgery.com/contactus

This book is not intended as a substitute for the medical advice of physicians. The reader should regularly consult a physician in matters relating to his/her health.

Print ISBN: 978-0-578-55363-4

eBook ISBN: 978-0-578-56231-5

# Testimonials

"This man is more than a surgeon. He is an artist! I would never let another doctor do anything on me. If you want better-than-expected results, go to Dr. Youssef."

—Kim P., Chino, CA

"Dr. Youssef is a doctor that I would entrust my mother with. Furthermore, I believe the art of being a great cosmetic surgeon is to do something to the patient and not make it obvious that something was done. You know something is different about someone, but you can't really put your finger on what it is. That's what Dr. Youssef does, he makes an improvement without being obvious."

—Seong Y., Los Angeles, CA

"I had such an amazing experience with Younique. Dr. Youssef and his staff were so thorough and comforting throughout my entire time with them. My results are incredible. I can't recommend them more!"

—Jessica P., Palmdale, CA

"Dr. Youssef is incredible. I've been going to him for years now. In fact, I even fly in from out of town to visit him. Now several of my friends are flying in to see him from multiple states as well as LA. I wouldn't go to anyone else. He is an expert all around. His office staff is wonderful too. They all take their time and listen. I never feel rushed I really can't say enough good things."

—Sarah C., Los Angeles, CA

"I came across Dr. Mark Youssef on accident, and from my first introduction I was sold. He is an amazingly genuine man who not only has mastered his craft, but makes you at ease in the most intense of situations. His staff is unlike many cosmetic surgery offices. They are *not* snooty or rude, and they treat you like family. He is a true artist."

—Carla W., Beverly Hills, CA

"I am the biggest cry baby when it comes to *any* kind of pain—Dr. Youssef is the only person I know who really makes me feel better! His kind words and patience with all my whimpering/whining during any procedure just makes me feel better."

—Suzie O., Santa Monica, CA

"I have been seeing Dr. Youssef for years now and despite his booming practice and celebrity-level practice, Dr. Youssef has remained down to earth, caring, extremely personable, and as patient as when I first met him! He is a phenomenal physician and you can trust him to help you achieve the best results possible! He and his staff treat you extremely warmly and are very helpful. There are not enough stars to rate him, as he surpasses any scale of excellence. I would recommend him whole heartedly!"

—J. P. , Los Angeles, CA

"What a wonderful experience I had with Dr. Youssef and the entire staff. Dr. Youssef is so humble (which is rare), and funny, and a wonderful person. It was such a positive experience. The staff was extremely brilliant and really wonderful making me feel like part of a family. Dr. Youssef knew exactly what I needed. He actually listened to what I wanted, offered suggestions, and I cannot tell you what a brilliant job he did! The follow-up was thorough and it really felt like everyone there was extremely invested in my experience being the best one possible. I would recommend this establishment to people considering plastic surgery who don't ever want to look like someone who had plastic surgery, but rather the best most natural version of themselves. I'd give more than five stars if I could!"

—Pamela H., Boulder, CO

"Dr. Youssef is absolutely fantastic. He was absolutely terrific. He has a very good bedside manner and listens to you and what you need. He's not afraid to say, "no you don't need that" when other doctors will push things on you. I would highly recommend Dr. Youssef and his staff to anyone."

—K B., Los Angeles, CA

"Dr. Youssef is awesome! I was referred to him by a friend after another Beverly Hills plastic surgeon messed me up big time. Yes, a Beverly Hills plastic surgeon! Dr. Youssef is so gentle, patient, caring, professional, and so down to Earth. He fixed up the mess that the other surgeon left. I feel safe and trust him thoroughly with the information that he has provided me with. I have also referred several friends to him—they all rave about him. I would go back to him in a heartbeat for any plastic surgery needs."

—Cynthia C., Los Angeles, CA

"The most important factors for me were that he was very knowledgeable, professional, and he really cares about you as a patient. He wanted to make sure that all my concerns would be addressed to make the result even better. He took pictures and asked about all my concerns before suggesting anything."

—Alyona K., Los Angeles, CA

"Dr. Youssef is amazing! Generally, I prefer female doctors, but Dr. Youssef is the exception. He is kind, patient, gentle, knowledgeable, and an excellent listener. His bedside manner is both comforting and professional. He patiently listened to my concerns and didn't make me feel rushed. I asked a lot of questions about products and services, and not once did he try to upsell me.

I really appreciated that he gave me all the information without pushing anything. My results were exactly what I wanted! I'm a perfectionist with high standards. I am not easy to please. However, Dr. Youssef exceeded my expectations. I will definitely be back to see him!"

—Alli A., West Hollywood, CA

"I had work done by Dr. Youssef and *he is amazing*! He's so sweet and really makes you feel comfortable even if it's your first time! I love him. I love the vibe, and the view is sooo amazing that you feel so calm and relaxed there!"

—Cesia A., Santa Clarita, CA

"Dr. Mark Youssef and his entire Younique staff are the absolute best—so welcoming, fun, and caring. The wonderful staff combined with the beautiful Santa Monica ocean front view makes you feel relaxed the moment you walk in the door."

—Emily S., Beverly Hills, CA

"The moment you walk in, everyone is calming and nurturing. They have a soothing wait area with beverages overlooking the beach. This place is top drawer."

—Michelle M., Santa Monica, CA

"Not only is the staff knowledgeable and professional, they are caring and understanding to boot. On top of the great care, the office is beautiful and comfortable, and the staff is present and personable. It's a luxury to visit Younique!"
—Maureen B., Redondo Beach, CA

"I am the happiest I've ever been in my life, and I can't thank Dr. Mark and his staff enough for my happiness. I am writing this review hoping it will help every perfectionist girl like me who will only trust the very best doctor out there.

When I look back, I can say that it's unbelievable how an operation that doesn't sound very pleasant to most was made to be such a fun experience for me by Dr. Mark and his incredibly wonderful team. Each and every individual who works with Dr. Mark is an amazing member of a genuinely caring team. There wasn't even one small moment I felt the slightest bit worried. Everybody involved was a confident and skilled professional. I received calls from Dr. Mark and his team every day after the surgery monitoring my process, letting me know they were available if need be, and assuring me that I was doing well. I had absolutely no complications after the operation. I went back to work six days after, and two weeks post-op I could not believe how good I looked. While Dr. Mark keeps saying that he just did his job, I know that not everybody does their job in the best, most meticulous, caring, and outstanding way."

—Vina M., Los Angeles, CA

# *This book is dedicated to:*

*Dr. Ivo Pitanguy*, the brilliant Brazilian plastic surgeon who pioneered the Brazilian Butt Lift. His Innovation continues to touch and inspire surgeons around the world.

*My surgical mentors* who took the time to take me under their wings and teach me the "art" of cosmetic surgery. These mentors changed my life by passing on their knowledge, talent, and passion. I hope to one day do the same for the next generation of surgeons. I am truly standing "on the shoulders of giants."

*My dear parents* who sacrificed their lives to come to this great country. Thank you for instilling in me the ingredients of success: dedication, perseverance, and passion. You always taught by example and told me to never give up on my dreams! I would not be where I am today without you.

# Table of Contents

Testimonials ............................................................ iii

Foreword: Beauty is Power by Dr. Miami ............ 1

Introduction: Your Body, Your Choice ................. 8

Chapter One: How Trends Have Popularized the Brazilian Butt Lift............................................. 14

    The Art of the Brazilian Butt Lift................... 15

    The Move Toward Natural ............................. 18

    Evolution Agrees............................................ 20

Chapter Two: The Big Booty Trend .................... 24

    How Music Has Influenced the Rise of the BBL...................................................... 27

    I Like Big Butts, and I Cannot Lie ................. 29

- Other Artists Follow: A Timeline .................. 31
- The New Ideal ................................ 36

Chapter Three: The Ideal Butt .......................... 38
- Three Features of An Ideal Butt .................... 42
- The Three Curves ............................... 43
- Four Types of Butts ............................. 44
- The A-shape .................................... 45
- The O-shape .................................... 46
- The H-shape .................................... 46
- The Inverted V-shape ............................ 47
- What's *Your* Ideal? ............................ 47

Chapter Four: Are You a Good Candidate for the Brazilian Butt Lift? .......................... 52
- General Health ................................. 53
- The Medical History and Physical Exam ........ 55
- The Photo ...................................... 58
- Weight ......................................... 60
- How to Calculate Your BMI ..................... 63
- Realistic Expectations ......................... 65

Chapter Five: Alternatives to the Brazilian

- Butt Lift .................................................. 70
- Implants .................................................. 71
  - Infection .............................................. 72
  - Capsular Contracture .......................... 73
  - Malposition of the Implant ................. 74
  - Pain After Surgery .............................. 74
- Collagen Stimulating Injections or Filler Injections ........................................ 75
- Beware of Black Market Butt Enhancements ........................................... 76
- Skin Tightening Lasers ............................ 79
- Other Options .......................................... 80

Chapter Six: Preparing for Your Surgery ........... 82
- The Happiness Curve .............................. 85
- Getting Ready for Surgery ....................... 89
  - Four Weeks Prior to Surgery ............... 89
  - Two Weeks Prior to Surgery ................ 90
  - One Week Prior to Surgery .................. 93
  - Your Caregiver ...................................... 93
  - Night Prior to and Morning of Surgery ...... 95

Chapter Seven: Post-Op and Recovery.............100

   Days One and Two..................................101

   Weeks One and Two................................106

      Physical Activity...............................107

      Cleanliness........................................108

      Fluids and Diet..................................109

      Smoking.............................................110

      Sleeping..............................................110

      Sitting Down......................................111

      Medications.......................................112

   Week Three............................................113

   Weeks Four and Five.............................115

   Weeks Six through Eight.......................117

   Additional Precautions During Recovery 117

   Possible Risks of the BBL......................118

Chapter Eight: What Happens to My
BBL Over Time?...............................................121

   The First and Second Change...............122

   The Lifetime of the BBL........................123

   Maintaining Your Shape........................126

The Bottom Line .............................................. 128

Chapter Nine: Team Work Makes
the Dream Work............................................ 130

The Experience ............................................. 131

Staying in Touch............................................ 133

I Promise to Put You...Second! ...................... 137

Our Specialty.................................................. 140

Conclusion........................................................... 143

Appendix............................................................. 145

The Brazilian Butt Lift FAQs......................... 145

Preparing For Your Surgery: At a Glance ...... 153

Pre-Operative Shopping List ........................ 159

Post-Operative Instructions ......................... 162

Medications to Avoid.................................... 168

# FOREWORD:
# Beauty is Power
# by Dr. Miami

Beauty is power. What does it mean to be powerful? It means being able to have people do things for you and living your life immersed in confidence. There are several strategies and resources you can use to become more powerful—how nice you are, how wealthy you are, how smart you are, and, yes, even how attractive you are. These are all levers of power people use to get through their lives and their days. In her book *Erotic Capital: The Power of Attraction in the Boardroom and the Bedroom*, renown sociologist Catherine Hakim discusses how erotic capital is as real as social capital or money capital in today's society.

As a cosmetic surgeon, I am in the business of empowering my patients with enhanced beauty and attractiveness. The more attractive you make yourself, the more confident you feel and the more powerful you are. Having extra confidence allows you to speak when you might not have otherwise felt comfortable enough to speak, or to apply for a job you might not have felt comfortable applying for. It changes how you interact with people, and that alone can change your life in significant ways.

Beauty *is* power.

For this reason, plastic surgery can be incredibly empowering. Until the discovery, invention, and perfection of plastic surgery, people were stuck with the bodies they were born with—for good or for bad. With the advancement of plastic surgery, however, people have the option to tweak the things that nature gave them in order to improve upon those things that you cannot really fix in the gym.

The Brazilian Butt Lift is a perfect example of

this. The BBL completely transforms your body's shape in a way you wouldn't be able to otherwise. There's no mechanism, no equipment, and no exercise you can do in the gym that is going to simultaneously narrow your waist and make your hips curvier. That just does not exist. There is no muscle on the hip there, so the only way to get that hourglass shape, if you're not born with it, is the BBL. This is a straightforward procedure in which we liposuction the fat from the areas you do not want it and put it in the places you do.

Plastic surgery allows you to take control not just of the things you eat, how much you work out, and how healthy you are on the inside—but of how you actually look in your clothing and how you feel when you present yourself to other people. The curvy look is ideal to much of today's society, and now you don't have to win the genetic lottery to get it. You can get it with the BBL. You can *choose* your ideal.

Some people have this idea—and it is an old-fashioned way of thinking that has fortunately been changing over the last two decades—that plastic surgery is cheating. They say, "You should just be natural and stay the way God made you." Really? Because I would argue that we never look at anything else in life that way. We do not say, "You are born naked, so stay naked!" Nobody says you shouldn't go to the doctor to have surgery when your appendix is inflamed for the sake of staying "all natural" and keeping your body the way it is. We do not demand that we should all live in caves because living in houses is too pretentious. No—we celebrate our opportunities and abilities to improve—and to correct—what nature gave us. Plastic surgery is just an extension of that.

The old mindset is a backwards way of thinking, and it certainly does not lead to progress or more human happiness. The flipside, of course, is that you do not want to be obsessed with plastic surgery and make it an addiction. Like all things, there is a time and place for everything. But for the right person at the right time in their lives and for the right reasons, plastic surgery can be a blessing.

I understand, however, that there can be some personal hurdles you need to overcome before you're ready to take this step. I have had plastic surgery myself, so I intimately understand the transformation people experience as they move through the "before" and "after" phases. I understand that the idea of physically altering yourself can be very intimidating. If for no other reason, the idea of surgery alone can be a little scary.

When you decide it's time, you'll go through the formalities of asking questions, finding a doctor, and making an appointment. From there, however, you must lead with your heart. *Choose* a doctor with whom you feel safe and comfortable. I cannot emphasize that enough. Plastic surgery requires you to bare your soul a little bit. It takes a lot of trust and vulnerability to get naked in front of a stranger and ask him to hold your insecurities. These can be huge psychological hurdles to overcome just to get to the point of getting through your initial consultation. From there, you will have so many questions about the surgery itself. There may be a lot of mystery to you about what goes on in the operating room, how the procedure is done, and what happens after. This can be intimidating, too.

These hurdles make a book like this and a doctor like Dr. Mark Youssef invaluable. This book thoroughly explains the BBL process in detail, which will answer your questions and help you overcome some of your fears. It makes the procedure more accessible and understandable for someone going through—or considering going through—this alteration. The more you learn, the more you know; and the more you know, the more powerful you are and the less fearful you become.

I am especially delighted that Dr. Mark Youssef is the one who chose to write this book. I know Dr. Youssef to be a kind, compassionate, and caring doctor. A good bedside manner is one of the most important qualities you need to look for in your surgeon. I think this is true in plastic surgery more than in any other specialty. Dr. Youssef excels at connecting with his patients and fulfilling what they want. Some surgeons have a "cookie cutter" mindset with a "You are getting what *I* want" attitude. Dr. Youssef is the opposite of this. He sincerely listens to each person who comes into his office. The importance of this trait cannot be understated.

The BBL is the most in-demand, most popular plastic surgery right now around the world—the US, South America, Asia, Europe, Australia, all over—as far as year over year growth. Whereas there have been roughly the same number of tummy tucks, rhinoplasties, and breast augmentations performed, the BBL has been almost doubling year over year for the last five or six years. With the increasing demand, however, I feel there are not enough quality surgeons out there. If you find one with experience and good bedside manner and who can deliver the results you want, you should definitely put him in your Rolodex and hold on to him because he is one of the few good surgeons out there.

I am honored to introduce this book, written by this particular doctor, to the world. I know how it feels when you look in the mirror and you see yourself a certain way. Everybody has an image of themselves in their minds. And as of right now, you're holding the power to change that image—and to change your life.

Best of wishes to you all,
Dr. Miami
a.k.a. Michael Salzhauer, MD

# INTRODUCTION
## *Your Body, Your Choice*

Judy walks into my office and takes a seat across from me. She is holding a tissue that she's twisting over and over again. Her posture is rigid. She will barely make eye contact with me. I start to ask her questions about her goals—why is she interested in a Brazilian Butt Lift?

Her eyes fill with tears and she looks down at the strangled tissue. "I've always been ridiculed and picked on because of my butt. In high school, my nickname was 'Flat Booty Judy'. It doesn't matter what I do, and trust me, I've tried everything. Everything! It doesn't matter how much I work out, or what herbs I take, or what foods I eat. I've never been able to wear the bathing suits I want to wear, and I've never felt comfortable going to pool parties or to the beach." Her shoulders slump. "I feel so powerless."

I can see the pain in her expression. I reach out and gently touch her hand. "I'm sorry you've had so much hurt and disappointment over this, Judy. I promise it won't always feel this way."

As we move into the exam portion of our visit, she pauses and takes a deep breath before removing her clothing. She squeezes her eyes closed and fresh tears spill down her cheeks. "You see what I mean?" she says. "My legs are basically connected straight into my back. I have no butt at all."

After the exam, we sit down to discuss her options. Her body type is perfect for this procedure! She's not too heavy, she's not too thin. I explain to her that we will gather some of the extra fat from her problem areas—her abdomen, love handles, and upper back—and relocate that fat into her buttocks in order to fill them out. I show her pictures of some of her options so she can determine which shape she likes best. She leafs through the pictures I've spread out on my desk and a smile spreads across her face. She looks up and makes direct eye contact with me.

"You can do this?" she asks as she points to an after picture of one of my patients. "My butt can look like this?"

"Yes, of course. Your body type is perfect for that. I think it's a great shape for you."

She beams at me, then studies the picture again. She closes her eyes, and I wonder if she's visualizing her near future.

Three months after her surgery, I find a letter on my desk with her return address. Inside is a small note and a 4x6 picture of Judy. The note reads, "This is the butt I've always wanted. Thank you!" I look at the picture and see her standing on the beach in a bright red swim suit. The most beautiful thing in the photo is her big, confident smile.

I slip the picture into my desk drawer, then open the door for my next consult.

\*\*\*

As a cosmetic surgeon, I am in the business of empowering my patients. You don't get to choose the body you are born with. However, you definitely get a say about the body you choose to live in.

I know there are people in your life who are

supportive of your decision to consider cosmetic surgery. But I also know those aren't the only voices that surround you. It may be your mom, your best friend, your partner, or any number of people who sincerely love you, who are begging you to change your mind.

While I appreciate their intention to show you their unconditional love, and you can see that for what it is, you must also understand that this is not the kind of decision you should ever make for other people. Only you know what it's like to live inside of your skin. You're the only one who has to. If you're taking a look around and thinking you'd like to make some improvements, then that is your right, and yours alone.

The opposite is also true. Maybe you picked up this book because a partner or a friend is pressuring you to make some enhancements. If that's the case, I encourage you to close this book right now and forget we ever met. Please, don't ever make these kinds of changes for someone else. Your body is sacred, and it is yours. Don't ever sign the deed over to another human.

When women lose sight of this, the result is usually pain. And I mean that both figuratively and literally. Consider some of the negative trends we've seen throughout the world's history, and even today. Foot binding, for example, was a Chinese practice that became popular during the Song dynasty (960-1279) and lasted for hundreds of years.[1] Women and female infants were subjected to the excruciating practice of breaking the bones in their feet so that it was curled up to fit into a tiny shoe. The smaller the woman's foot, the more attractive it was considered to be. That procedure went far outside the body's natural proclivity toward beauty to create something unnatural and painful. Women lived with life-long disabilities and deformities as a result.

Who came up with something so barbaric as a standard for beauty? It certainly wasn't the infant. That was a result of other people making choices for the individual.

The purpose of this book is to empower you with the information and science you need in order to determine if the Brazilian Butt-Lift is a good fit for *you*.

I promise that surgery is not as extreme as some of your critics may think. It's not much different from braces, Lasik eye correction, or piercing your ears. These are all physical alterations to your appearance in order to improve what God gave you. What you and I do together in my office is no different. We are simply making some improvements to what you were born with in order to improve the quality of your life. Do I think you need a butt lift in order to be happy? No, not at all. I think you need to be happy in order to be happy, and if you've decided that the butt lift is the way to make that happen, then so be it.

I think of my office as a kind of cosmetic Disneyland—the happiest place on Earth. Indeed, it is a place where dreams can come true.

Even yours.

---

[1] See https://en.wikipedia.org/wiki/Foot_binding.

# CHAPTER ONE
## *How Trends Have Popularized the Brazilian Butt Lift*

*Life imitates art far more than art imitates life.*
~ Oscar Wilde

The space I share with my patients is a vulnerable, intimate one where they confide in me their most private desires, and then I do my best to make their dreams come true. This takes more than training, skill, and ability. It requires a touch of magic. When I go to work as a cosmetic surgeon, I think of myself as an artist more than I do a physician or surgeon. Yes, I am those other things as well, but I can't *just* be those things. A great cosmetic surgeon must have an artist's eye. I must understand proportions, curves, and how to use the full potential of my canvas. I capture my patient's vision and then I sculpt and create it with what I have to start with.

This takes more than just "freeing David from marble." Artists who are starting with a piece of stone or a block of wood have an advantage because they're starting with something that can be sculpted into anything. As a cosmetic surgeon on the other hand, I can only work with what the patient brings to me. My artistry often requires architecture. My only option is to work with the patient's existing skin tissue, their elasticity, their genetic body habitus, and then I go from there.

## The Art of the Brazilian Butt Lift

The Brazilian Butt Lift (BBL) is no different. I have to rely on my imagination, skill, and artistry in order to get you as close to where you want to be without compromising the intrinsic beauty of the rest of your body. It's not just about what we're adding or taking away, but also the proportion of what we're adding or taking away. This is not just a localized procedure. It is a whole-body procedure and I must be considerate of the proportions of the rest of your body as well. It's not just about what we want your butt to look like, but what we want your butt to look like on your specific body.

This is extremely important because this is what makes your BBL a classic improvement—one that will be just as socially appealing thirty years from now as it is today. When we lose sight of the importance of proportions and begin to work against your body's natural potential, that is when extreme trends arise that may not serve you in the long term nor will they stand the test of time.

And trends like these do make an appearance from time to time.

In the seventies and eighties, just a few short decades ago, the popular trend was to get very large breast implants. Stars like Dolly Parton and Pamela Anderson are icons of this trend. The bigger the boobs the better. But over time, people began to realize that even though that practice was not nearly as harmful as foot binding, there were still negative long-term side effects. The heavy breasts caused chronic back pain, and the large implants caused skin thinning and stretch marks on the breasts. The practice of putting large foreign objects into the body so far outside of women's natural proportions affected the way women stood and walked, their ability to run, and their basic quality of life. These are some of the consequences of stepping away from the whole-body perspective when making localized augmentations.

The Brazilian Butt Lift is a more natural procedure with fewer risks of long-term side effects. Instead of using implants, you are simply transferring fat from one area of your body into another. Instead of introducing foreign materials into your body, you're working with your body's natural resources and proportions. It's something you can love and keep for the rest of your life. There are no long-term side effects or fear of living in pain or discomfort.

## The Move Toward Natural

More and more, today's cosmetic trends are moving toward celebrating our bodies' natural potential for beauty. Cosmetic surgery is still a booming industry, but where people were once undergoing dramatic alterations to the point that they were no longer recognizable, now patients are opting for less dramatic alterations that enhance the attractiveness of what is already there. Make no mistake—you are already beautiful. My job is not to transform you into a stranger, but to help you step more fully into the potential you already have. Kenny Rogers, Mickey Rourke, Dolly Parton, and Joan Rivers are the poster children of a generation of cosmetic trends that we are now abandoning. Today, you almost have to hold most celebrities' before and after pictures side-by-side in order to detect the subtle differences that have enhanced their attractiveness.

This movement away from extreme augmentations is part of the overall backlash to the Photoshop culture. Everybody knows that any model, female figure, or celebrity that is put on the cover of a magazine is photoshopped. Photoshop has been key in creating the gold standard of how we perceive people and how we strive to emulate "perfection." Eating disorders have increased in epidemic proportions because these visuals on television and magazines are promoting unrealistic ideals of beauty. It's reported that 35% to 57% of adolescent girls now practice extreme forms of dieting such as fasting, diet pills, crash dieting, self-induced vomiting, or laxatives.[1] Our society has been guilty of putting pressure on women to contort themselves into looking a certain way—to have no cellulite, have perfectly symmetrical eyes, long eyelashes, and the presence or absence of certain curves to their bodies. All of these things were artificially being tweaked with photoshop to the point that they weren't realistic, and it was the expectation that you should emulate these surreal standards.

Tina Fey says, "I find, the fancier the fashion magazine is, the worse the Photoshop. It's as if they are already so disgusted that a human has to be in the clothes, they can't stop erasing human features."

Over the past decade or two, especially as iconic, voluptuous superstars like Jennifer Lopez (J. Lo) have emerged onto the scene, we're seeing almost a backlash to this photoshop culture. People are saying, "Natural is beautiful. If you're a little curvy or have a big butt, you're fine. If you're a little heavy, it's OK. You're beautiful." You can see this being reflected in movements like Dove's campaign to show real women—those with average and over-sized body types—that you don't have to be photoshopped stick-thin to be beautiful.

## Evolution Agrees

One of the reasons this trend is likely to last is because it is so closely linked to our most ancient drives and instincts. Even though you will find different standards of beauty across the world and throughout history, there are some ideals that are innate in us. Subconsciously, the human eye sees symmetry as beauty. In other words, when a woman's face is symmetrical, when her breasts are symmetrical, when her buttocks is symmetrical, she is considered to be more beautiful. The closer the left side of our body looks like your right, and vice versa, the more others subconsciously view you as beautiful because, in the human mind, symmetry is closer to perfect. There's a lot of beauty in a nice, round symmetrical buttocks, like bubble butts, because it is so symmetrical. You don't have a lot of shadows and there are no indents. The upper part looks like the lower part, and the outer part looks like the inner part. Everything looks homogenous and symmetrical.

These aren't arbitrary standards, but standards that have helped to perpetuate our species for millions of years. I believe one of the reasons we are so drawn to larger bottoms is because evolution has trained our brains to identify signs of fertility and strength. When a woman has wider hips and a more voluptuous buttocks, science tells us that this gives the subconscious impression of more fertility and a better ability to bear children, which makes her more attractive to men. The same is true with breasts. Subconsciously, we know breasts are for breast feeding, and even though it is not directly correlated, subconsciously our human brain associates larger breasts with a better ability to nurse, and therefore help to perpetuate a healthy and strong human population. Even our basic common sense can surmise that a strong, healthy woman is more likely to have strong, healthy children. So, our appreciation for the big booty goes back further than J. Lo and the Kardashians. It goes all the way back to our first human ancestors who were primed for survival. We have come a long way since then, but the same mechanics are still operating in our brains today.

In 1995, Swiss biologist Claus Wedekind conducted a study called "the sweaty T-shirt study." Besides the waist hip-ratio giving a subconscious view of fertility, the sweaty t-shirt study found that women are attracted to men with a certain sweat and men are attracted to women with a certain sweat, but it is not the same for everyone. When a woman is attracted to a certain type of sweat from a man, genetically that man has a complementary genetic makeup to hers. In other words, the woman's genetics plus the sweaty man's sweat to which she is attracted will create a better DNA offspring than somebody whose sweat they are unattracted to. In other words, our DNA actually forces us to be attracted to people who would allow us to have better genetic offspring.[2]

This shift toward celebrating our natural

bodies is reflected in what is happening in our pop culture, and our current pop culture is a reflection of what is happening in our trends. They have been feeding into each other until today's public now more easily acknowledges the desirability of a larger backside.

---

[1] Boutelle, Neumark-Sztainer, Story, & Resnick, 2002; Neumark-Sztainer & Hannan, 2001; Wertheim et al., 2009.

[2] See https://en.wikipedia.org/wiki/Claus_Wedekind.

## CHAPTER TWO
## *The Big Booty Trend*

When the rampant rumor started that J. Lo had insured her backend for as much as $1 billion, the public didn't even blink. Why? Because who *wouldn't* insure such a valuable asset? (No pun intended.) That is how much we as a society have come to revere the curvier female frame.

We are deeply influenced by what we see in media. From the time we are born, humans tend to model what they see. This is why fashion trends are such a viral phenomenon. The magazines and music surrounding us affects our beliefs and desires. Media psychology is now an official subspecialty in the field of psychology and is a growing field of interest. This acute influence of media on our perspectives is why most of my BBL patients are between the ages of 18 and 45. Those are the years we are most interested in, and influenced by, popular fashions and social media.

Today, women in their young adult years don't question the beauty of a fuller behind. They are entering adulthood as this cultural trend continues to hit its peak. Trend setters like J. Lo, the Kardashians, and Iggy Azalea are household names to most women today.

However, women at the far end of this age spectrum are witnessing the historical shifts happening in real time. They fell in love with J. Lo when she was just "Jenny from the block," and recognize her as the queen she is in leading the "big-bum movement." As one writer recently phrased it on vh1.com, "Bow down to the queen who was twerking when Iggy was still in grade school."[1]

Just before the turn of the century, J. Lo simultaneously emerged into mainstream media as both a movie star and a musician. In 2000, she broke the Internet with the jaw-dropping dress she wore to the Grammys as she dangled from P. Diddy's arm.

In 2001, she became the first woman in the United States to have both a number one album and a number one film at the same time.[2] She was everywhere. And so was her message—you don't have to be rail thin to be sexy. In 1998, Details magazine named her the "Sexiest Woman of the Year." *Vanity Fair* described her derriere as a cultural icon.[3] In many ways, she redefined the standard and gracefully accepted the responsibility she carried as a role model.

In 2001, she became a triple threat when she launched her clothing and accessory company, J. Lo By Jennifer Lopez. Her clothing line was a business move as much as it was a cultural statement. She expressed her feelings that the voluptuous woman was under-represented in fashion trends, which was why her line intentionally catered to women of all shapes and sizes.

What we are seeing in media today is influencing the popularity of the Brazilian Butt Lift. We are being inundated with images of Kim Kardashian, Nikki Minaj, J. Lo, Iggy Azalea, Sofia Vergara, and other models of this movement. What they are showing us is that big bottoms are beautiful, and the public is responding. In 2012, it was reported that there had been a 235 percent increase in buttocks augmentations in the previous decade.[4] While this feature is a more natural hallmark of female Latino and African American body types, it is refreshing to see this kind of diversity being celebrated throughout today's culture. Historically, it was the white female's body type being put on a pedestal as the standard for all. In the twenties, the white flapper culture promoted flat backends. In the fifties, women like Marilyn Monroe and Liz Taylor set the standard for curvier body types. In the nineties, we saw super model Naomi Campbell sporting curves, but on the other end of the spectrum we still had super models like Kate Moss and Elle Macpherson popularizing the rail-thin body type with almost no butt to speak of. However, to our credit, since 2010, many of our icons have come from a diverse ethnic background, which has largely been fueled by modern music.

## How Music Has Influenced the Rise of the BBL

Music has a dramatic impact on us, both individually and as a society. It has always been this way.

According to John Blacking, a renowned ethnomusicologist, music is not something that is taught, but is instead something that is brought out in each of us.[5] Music is part of our human inheritance. Think of the last time you were cooing at a baby or saw someone else engaging in that kind of "baby talk." It's no coincidence that what we commonly call baby talk seems to be universal. Scientifically, this common sing-song voice is known as infant-directed-speech (IDS).[6] This musical form of communication is used cross-culturally by men and women, and by parents and non-parents alike. It's wired into us.

Steven Mithen, a professor of Archaeology at the University of Reading, says in his book *The Singing Netherlands*, "We talk like this because human infants demonstrate an interest in, and sensitivity to, the rhythms, tempos, and melodies of speech long before they are able to understand the meanings of words…. [I]t appears that the neural networks for language are built upon, or replicate, those for music." This shows that music has a developmental priority over language. Parents are quick to pick up on this, even if it is unconsciously.

IDS is used (successfully) to communicate intent.[7]

All of this tells us that music is one of our most ancient and intrinsic languages. It is no wonder that it has so much power to shape who we are. One anonymous author said it well with these words: "Music is so influential on the brain that the type you listen to actually has the ability to change the way you think and look at the world." It is the most appropriate tool for telling stories and expressing our deepest desires because it amplifies the words it carries. The story that today's music is telling us is that curvy and big is beautiful.

## I Like Big Butts, and I Cannot Lie

Sir Mix-A-Lot was one of the most iconic musicians to set the stage for this story. He aggressively pushed back against the Photoshop culture in 1992 with his famous song, "Baby Got Back." The lyrics state, "I'm tired of magazines sayin' flat butts are the thing... Yeah, baby, when it comes to females, *Cosmo* ain't got nothin' to do with my selection. Thirty-six twenty-four thirty-six... So *Cosmo* says you're fat, well I ain't down with that 'cause your waist is small and your curves are kickin'."

Sir Mix-A-Lot was one of the first artists in popular song to tell us that Photoshop is unnecessary, in fact, it's a bad thing, and we don't need to emulate unrealistic, skinny people who often don't even look like that in real life. In an interview for the "Where Are They Now" segment on the Oprah Winfrey Network in 2016, he said he got the idea for the song after watching a beer commercial where the girls were shaped "like stop signs." He said:

> "That's where I realized, 'You know what, there is another [kind of] beautiful that for some reason isn't being talked about much.' And I wanted to talk about it. ... I didn't want women to look at *Cosmo* as the goal. I wanted to shift what the goal was. Don't look at *Cosmo* and say, 'I gotta get that physique so they'll put me in pictures.' Don't worry about them! Baby, you are beautiful, you are gorgeous, you can do what you want to do."[8]

The public received the message with open arms. The song spent five weeks at number one, was the second-best selling song of the year, sold over two million copies, and is still making waves today, as can be seen with Nikki Minaj's recent tribute to the song with her single "Anaconda." The release and reception of "Baby Got Back" dramatically affected our beliefs and views on desirable proportions. It opened people's eyes to a totally new way of looking at a woman who had a big butt. It was no longer a negative thing. He almost flip-flopped the perception. Instead of the idea that we have to digitally carve women into a skinny, size-6 person, we should like curvy women because that is more natural.

## Other Artists Follow: A Timeline

Sir Mix-A-Lot was the engine that pulled a big train. Floods of artists picked up his message and amplified it, and the trend continues today. Here are some of the most iconic songs and moments that have paved the way to today's artists and the growing trend of the Brazilian Butt Lift.

**1998:** "Back That Azz Up," recorded by Juvenile and featuring Mannie Fresh and Lil Wayne.

Wikipedia describes this song as "an explicit exploration of the same themes as Sir Mix-A-Lot's "Baby Got Back."

**1999:** "Thong Song," recorded by Sisqó.

The music video was a sensation and is credited for the new trend of "booty" videos that followed. Sisqó did a remake of this song and video in 2017, showcasing its classic appeal to fans.

**2000:** "Bootylicious," recorded by Destiny's Child.

This wasn't the first time the word "Bootylicious" was used to describe a sexually attractive female, but this is the song that made the term so popular and wide spread, which led to the word being officially recognized and added to the Oxford English Dictionary in 2004.[9]

**2003:** "Salt Shaker," recorded by The Yin Yang Twins and featuring Lil Jon and The East Side Boyz.

**2004:** "My Humps," recorded by the Black Eyed Peas.

This song celebrates a woman's curves.

**2005:** "Shake That," recorded by Eminem and featuring Nate Dogg.

**2008:** "Low," recorded by Flo Rida and featuring T-Pain.

A memorable song in which the featured female in the song gives "that big booty a smack." This was the most downloaded single of the decade (2000-2010) and was the longest-running number-one single the year it was released.[10] It helped popularize Apple Bottom jeans, which were designed to celebrate and emphasize the apple-shaped behind.

**2012:** "Bubble Butt," recorded by Major Lazer and featuring Bruno Mars, 2 Chainz, Tyga, and Mystic.

This song celebrates the bubble butt. The music video comically shows women with small backends being featured as stiff and negative, then having hoses attached to them to inflate their butts, followed by them cutting loose and dancing. The visuals here infer how your life can improve by swapping out a small back end for a bubble butt. This is a song that a lot of cosmetic surgeons play in the operating room while they're performing the BBL procedure.

**2012:** "Twerk It," recorded by Busta Rhymes and featuring Nicki Minaj.

**2013:** Miley Cyrus brings twerking front and center.

On August 25, 2013, just a few months after the release of Busta Rhymes' "Twerk It" (recorded in 2012), Miley Cyrus broke the Internet with her controversial performance at the MTV Video Music Awards. The performance garnered 306,100 tweets per minute and became the subject of a massive public dialogue. Although twerking was not new, it was new to white America and considered very extreme for its time. However, her appropriating twerking into white culture created a bridge between cultures that paved the way for even white Americans to embrace the big booty trend.

**2013:** "Wiggle," recorded by Jason Derulo and featuring Snoop Dogg.

**2014:** "All About That Bass," recorded by Meghan Trainor.

This song is a discussion about positive body image, regardless of your size. It is part of the dialogue surrounding the current trend toward a more curvaceous and natural beauty. Some of the lyrics include, "If you got beauty beauty just raise 'em up 'cause every inch of you is perfect from the bottom to the top. Yeah, my momma she told me don't worry about your size. She says, boys they like a little more booty to hold at night." She, too, talks about the need to reject the Photoshop culture, which continues to amplify the themes in Sir Mix-A-Lot's iconic song twenty years earlier.

**2014:** "Booty," recorded by J. Lo, featuring Iggy Azalea.

As one of the most iconic celebrities that championed this trend in the early 2000s, J. Lo continues to spread the message that big is beautiful in this single with lyrics like, "Big, big booty, what you got a big booty. You're gorgeous. I mean you're fine. You're sexy, but most of all, you are just absolutely booty-full." The song features Iggy Azalea, who is another icon of the big-butt movement. The two artists sensualize how desirable it is to have a large backend.

**2014:** "Anaconda," recorded by Nikki Minaj.

Written and performed as a tribute to Sir Mix-A-Lot's "Baby Got Back," the song brings the movement full circle. In an interview with Billboard, Sir Mix-A-Lot said, "[W]hen I did 'Baby Got Back,' women with curves were not accepted. But that's a fact, they were not in the mainstream. We've come 180 degrees from that point. Not only is it accepted, but it's also expected...."

## The New Ideal

All of these songs and media icons have been monumental in shifting our culture's preferences and opening our eyes to the true measure of a woman's natural beauty. Today's fitness magazines, which once upon a time focused primarily on how to reduce the size of your backend, now regularly run features and provide tips on how to increase the size of your butt and make it more "bubble" shaped. Popular brands like Dove and Forever 21 are hiring more full-bodies models to market their products. The ideal butt is not being reinvented. It is finally being recognized, celebrated, and accepted cross-culturally.

I am grateful for the opportunity I have to take part in this worthwhile movement.

---

[1] Taylor Ferber, "Shame on You for Forgetting J. Lo Has the Original Best Butt" Web Article, 24 July 2017; http://www.vh1.com/news/37676/jennifer-lopez-has-original-best-butt/.

[2] See https://en.wikipedia.org/wiki/Jennifer_Lopez.

[3] See https://en.wikipedia.org/wiki/Jennifer_Lopez.

[4] 235 Percent increase, Meet the New LA Ideal.

[5] Steven Mithen, *The Singing Neanderthals* (Massachusetts: Harvard, 2006), 16.

[6] Steven Mithen, *The Singing Neanderthals* (Massachusetts: Harvard, 2006), 69.

[7] Steven Mithen, *The Singing Neanderthals* (Massachusetts: Harvard, 2006), 71.

[8] OWN TV, The Inspiration Behind Sir Mix-a-Lot's *Baby Got Back* (Where Are They Now); Youtube Video 7 July 2017; https://www.youtube.com/watch?v=wl5-O87felU.

[9] See https://en.wikipedia.org/wiki/Destiny's_Child.

[10] See https://en.wikipedia.org/wiki/Flo_Rida.

# CHAPTER THREE
## *The Ideal Butt*

So, what *is* the ideal butt? That is something for you to personally decide. So, the better question to really ask is, "What is the ideal butt for *you*?" The answer is going to be relative to your unique preferences and your body type. However, today's research and trends are definitely telling us that big is beautiful.

One study, *Redefining the Ideal Buttocks: A population analysis*, conducted a study with 1146 participants in order to determine what the ideal waist-hip ratio, or WHR, is in women (i.e. the most desirable butt size). This ratio is determined by dividing the waist measurement by the hip measurement.

The smaller the number, the bigger the butt is in proportion to the size of the waist. The reverse is also true. The bigger the number, the closer the size of the waist is to the size of the buttocks. For example, someone with a square buttocks and a square waist will have a higher WHR because their waist and their hip are not going to be very different, meaning the ratio will be closer to 1.

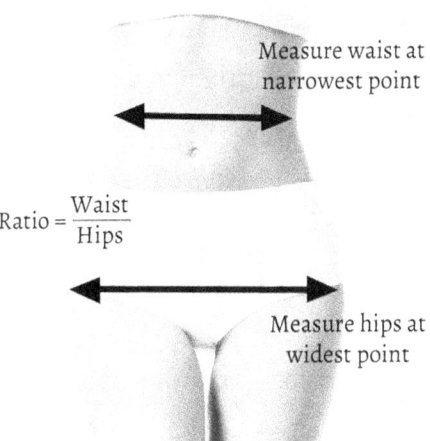

The study showed there has been a dramatic shift in what is considered ideal by today's standards. Historically, the ideal was a 0.7 ratio. Today, the ideal is a ratio of 0.60-0.65. That means people prefer rear ends that are 7-15 percent larger than the previous standard of beauty! The study's conclusion states the preference for these new ratios "indicate a more dramatic and 'curvier' new ideal, signaling an important preference paradigm shift." It's also interesting to note that there were no significant differences in preferences between respondent ages, genders, or ethnicities. This is a *universal* preference.[1]

This new standard is why we saw a 235 percent increase in the number of BBLs being done in the previous decade. If the ideal WHR suggests it's better to have a bigger butt in proportion to the size of your waist, then you are looking at either increasing the size of your butt or decreasing the size of your waist. Often, the BBL presents the opportunity for you to do both because we are often transferring fat from the abdomen waistline into the buttocks.

Even if the fat is coming from a different area, it's still a lot easier to increase the size of your backend than it is to augment the size of your waist. At some point, no matter how thin you are, genetically your waist can only be so small. Some women used to try to cheat the system by having surgery to remove their twelfth rib, also termed the floating rib, which is the lowest and closest rib to your waist. So, aside from extreme surgery, it is much easier to increase your hip and buttocks circumference than it is to decrease the size of your waist.

It is no surprise, then, that the celebrities most beloved for their booties fall into this ideal 0.6-0.65 WHR range—nor it is surprising that some of these women were not born with these beautiful backends.[2]

|  | Waist | Hips | Ratio |
|---|---|---|---|
| Coco Austin | 23 | 40 | 0.58 |
| Nicki Minaj | 26 | 45 | 0.58 |
| Iggy Azalea | 23 | 37 | 0.62 |
| Kim Kardashian | 26 | 40 | 0.65 |
| Beyoncé | 26 | 40 | 0.65 |
| Blac Chyna | 27 | 41 | 0.66 |
| J. Lo | 25 | 38 | 0.66 |
| Amber Rose | 25 | 38 | 0.66 |
| Rhianna | 24 | 36 | 0.67 |
| Pippa Middleton | 23 | 34 | 0.68 |
| Kimberley Walsh | 25 | 35 | 0.71 |
| Kelly Brook | 25 | 35 | 0.71 |
| Jessica Biel | 26 | 36 | 0.72 |

## Three Features of An Ideal Butt

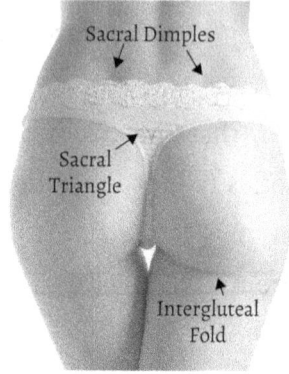

Your WHR gives a lot of information, but not a lot of details. Size is only part of what makes the aesthetic difference. In the diagram, you will see examples of the three features of an ideal butt—the details that we're looking for because they give us good anatomical landmarks. They are:

- **Sacral dimples:** These are the dimples right above the buttocks.
- **The sacral triangle:** This is the V-shaped crease formed at the top of the buttocks.
- **The intergluteal fold:** This is the little crease below the buttocks. This one is of special note. Ideally, you want that to be pretty short because if it is all the way across, it means the butt is droopy. The closer that crease is to your outer hip, the more your butt will sag.

## The Three Curves

When I assess the strategy for transforming what you have into your ideal butt, we are generally going to be looking at measurements of three specific curves, or arcs. The first curve is the one going from your lower back to your legs. The second curve goes from the outer hip to the butt crack. The third curve we want to consider is the arc going from the waist down to the outer hip—the outer arch. All three of these curves are important depending on what you want.

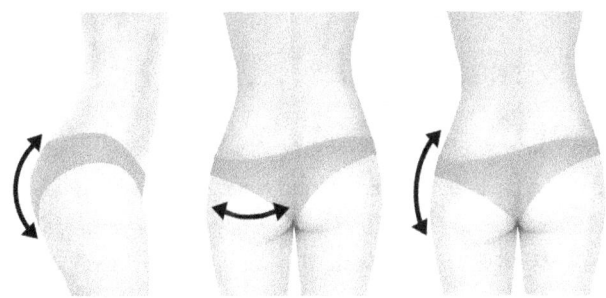

I am always asking, "What am I taking away? What do I need to leave?" What I leave behind is just as important as what I am taking away or adding. You already have a canvas for me to work with, and I want to make the transition from what you have to what you want as natural as possible.

For example, if you have a square butt "canvas," you're actually giving me a lot to work with. Simply removing the fat from those outer corners will automatically augment your shape to be rounder and more aesthetically pleasing without even adding any more fat. I simply need to remove the undesirable frame around the buttocks to reveal the hidden beauty within what you already have.

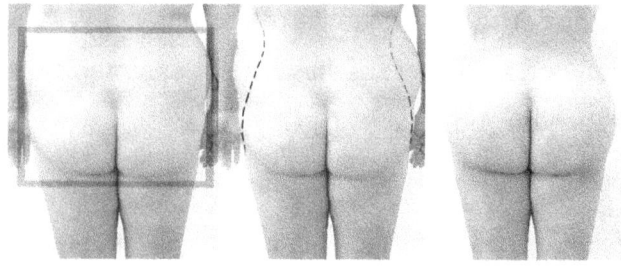

*Here's an example of one of our patients with an H-shaped butt that simply needed the "frame" of fat removed, as well as a little augmentation, to give her the look she wanted. the removal of the fat makes this result more dramatic than the augmentation alone.*

## Four Types of Butts

There are four predominant butt shapes, each of which present a different frame, or canvas, for me to work with. They are as follows:

- **The A-shape**, or upside-down heart
- **The O-shape**, or round, bubble butt
- **The H-shape**, or square
- **The V-shape**, or inverted triangle

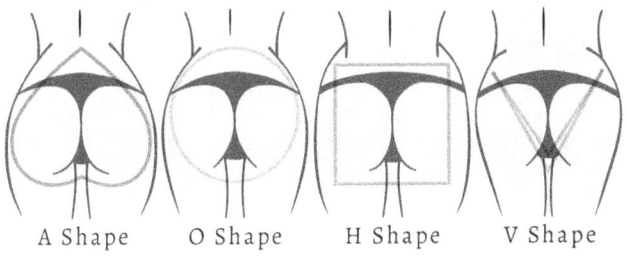

A Shape   O Shape   H Shape   V Shape

## The A-shape

The A-shape, also known as the upside-down heart or inverted pear shape, is considered to be the most feminine of all four types. In this instance, the waist has a more tapered look and the buttocks tends to widen below the hip bone, as the fat distribution is heavier in the lower half of the buttocks, giving it that upside-down heart shape. Oftentimes, this distribution of fat is hormonally related, as increased estrogen levels can sometimes create this shape. As women get older and move into menopause, estrogen levels decrease, which increases their fat storage around the midsection and abdominal area instead of the buttocks.

## The O-shape

Then we have the O-shaped, or round buttocks, which is what a lot of the songs in the previous chapter refer to as the bubble butt. Bubble butts are round, almost perfectly circular butts where the fat is distributed evenly around the cheeks, including the upper portion, like a balloon. Round butts are usually full and perky. This shape is fairly popular, as this is the shape we see on some of the hottest celebrities such as Kim Kardashian, Queen Bey, and J. Lo. This shape also tends to be seen in more muscular, athletic women due to the roundness of the gluteal muscles.

## The H-shape

The H-shape, also known as the square shape, is determined by the bone structure of the pelvis and the femur bones in the thighs. Usually, people are H-shaped because they have a genetic tendency to carry fat in their love handles, which increases the measurements of the waist and gives the woman more of a SpongeBob SquarePants look. If a woman wants a shapelier, rounder butt, the H-shape is creating a frame of too much fat around the buttocks, like we mentioned above.

## The Inverted V-shape

The V-shape, or inverted triangle, is most commonly seen in older women because estrogen levels tend to drop after menopause. As estrogen levels go down, the midsection starts to carry more fat and the buttocks starts to become flatter and less full, which starts to create a wider upper butt and a flatter, narrower lower butt, which creates that upside-down V shape. This shape usually lacks volume on the outer half and the lower buttocks.

## What's *Your* Ideal?

The truth is that there is no ideal, one-size-fits-all buttocks. You will have your own unique vision of what you want yours to reflect based on your preferences. Although the upside-down heart shape is currently most popular, you may prefer the more symmetrical bubble butt with larger or smaller measurements than someone else. Ultimately, each procedure comes down to the purpose of improving your butt by making it rounder and more lifted. Within those two categories, people have varying ideals.

Today, the majority of my BBL patients are Hispanic or African American, but celebrities like Miley Cyrus and Iggy Azalea are influencing white Americans to embrace this trend, too. Culturally, each patient is likely to have different expectations. If a Latino or African American patient goes up a size in their jeans after this procedure, they would consider the procedure a success. On the other hand, a Caucasian patient may be mortified if she had to buy larger pants.

Common sense tells us that cultural norms will influence our preferences, and science backs this up. Studies show that our perceptions of beauty are influenced by our geographic, ethnic, cultural, and demographic factors. One such study found that among surgeons who were asked to define the ideal buttocks size, "surgeons in Latin America preferred the largest buttocks, followed by surgeons in Asia, North America, and Europe, with non-Caucasians preferring larger buttocks than Caucasians."[3]

So, your ideal is as unique as you are.

As your surgeon, the most important thing I can do is to listen to what you want. As an artist, I will also counsel you on my recommendations for what is going to make your unique body most beautiful. This is where proportions come into play and are so vital. This is true for *any* procedure you may be having done. For instance, if you're getting a breast augmentation, you don't want to go too big or too small, and that "big" or "small" is largely going to be based on your other proportions. This is the best way to enhance what you already have and ensure it still looks natural. In addition, if someone does a normal augmentation in keeping with their natural proportions, the chances of them having complications or back pain or any sort of negative effects as a result of the procedure are minimal. The larger you go, the more likely you are to have issues down the road.

It's the same with the BBL procedure. If you have something that is a nice improvement with a normal-sized augmentation and good proportions to the rest of your body, then you have minimal risks ten to twenty years from now. However, if you have very large amounts of fat transferred, when you hit menopause and have a loss of elasticity, loss of collagen, and loss of firmness in your skin, there is a chance that extra fat can make your buttocks look a little bit droopy as gravity takes its toll. It won't be as round, or as firm, or look as good as it did when you were younger. This is why my professional and artistic recommendation is going to take into consideration things like your unique height, weight, bone structure, skin elasticity, how wide your shoulders are, and where you are genetically predisposed to carry fat.

For instance, some women say they want as much taken away from their thighs as possible. That sounds great in theory, but that's not something that's going to look good on every patient. It's not normal to have scrawny legs connected to a big butt on a skinny body. I don't want you to be a "butt on a stick." Part of the artistry is calculating how much to leave behind so that it looks normal. We don't want to leave anything with a defect or a void. Creating your ideal butt requires a plan, and these are all components of that plan.

That being said, if you want something that's a little bit more or a little bit less than what I recommend, I am here to serve you and will do everything in my power to make your dreams come true—whatever they are.

---

[1] "Redefining the Ideal Buttocks: A Population Analysis," PubMed.gov, 2017; https://www.ncbi.nlm.nih.gov/pubmed/27219230.

[2] "Bad luck, Kim: Coco Austin is queen of the rears... as we see how celebrities measure up in battle of the booties," 22 April 2014; https://www.dailymail.co.uk/femail/article-2610218/Rounder-rumps-celebrated-ten-celebrity-rears-featuring-Kim-Kardashian-Nicki-Minaj.html.

[3] American Society of Plastic Surgeons, (Ideal Buttock Size: A Sociodemographic Morphometric Evaluation, Volume 140, Number 1), 30e.

# CHAPTER FOUR
# *Are You a Good Candidate for the Brazilian Butt Lift?*

Are you a good candidate for the Brazilian Butt Lift? There are a few things that you need to be aware of before you decide if this procedure is right for you. Luckily, there is some wiggle room to some of the requirements, meaning that even if you aren't an ideal candidate today—based on your percentage of body fat or your smoking habits—those are fluid factors. In many cases, we can work together to prepare your body and your lifestyle for this procedure if you do not already qualify.

**Note:** This chapter is designed to give you a loose framework for what makes you an ideal candidate, but it is not meant to be a guide to an at-home assessment. There are factors unique to you and your body to be considered that will be more, or less, in your favor than you realize. A qualified physician is necessary for determining whether you are ready for this procedure.

## General Health

The main consideration for this procedure is your general level of health, both physically and mentally. You have to be pretty healthy to undergo this procedure because even though it is not major surgery, it's still invasive surgery that requires anesthesia and recovery time. We need to make sure that your body is currently in a state to be able to handle those things. I care about your results—however, I care about your health and safety more.

This isn't a huge concern for most of my BBL patients because they generally fall between the healthy ages of eighteen and forty-five. However, if you are a regular smoker or drinker, these habits could cause problems for you. Smoking and the regular consumption of alcohol can cause complications with the anesthesia and impede your healing process. You won't be disqualified from the procedure, but you will be required to refrain from these routines for a period of time leading up to the surgery. We will discuss this in more detail in *Chapter Six: Preparing For Your Surgery*.

We also want to be sensitive to your age. There isn't an age limit, but in general, if you're over the age of fifty, you will need to have medical clearance by your primary care physician and have an EKG performed, which is an assessment of the strength and condition of your heart. These steps keep you safe while you're going through the procedure and make sure you are healthy enough to undergo the anesthesia.

In addition, most physicians have a maximum weight cutoff because obese patients have an increased risk under anesthesia. (We will talk more about this below.)

## The Medical History and Physical Exam

Before I approve you for the BBL procedure, my staff and I will do our homework to determine whether you are a good fit. We will do a physical exam and get your basic health history in order to get a complete picture of any current medical conditions, chronic illnesses, past surgeries, or any sort of complications to anesthesia you've had in the past. We will talk about any allergies you might have to medications—specifically those medications we're going to use in the procedure. We will get information about what medications you're taking to confirm none of them interact with those we administer while you're under anesthesia.

We will collect your family's medical history, especially as it relates to anything that pertains to the body habitus, which is your physique or body build. For instance, many women come in and say their entire family is pear-shaped—everyone is really little on top with skinny arms, a tiny chest, and a flat stomach; and they all have really big, thick thighs. These are genetic things that we want to know about and try to compensate for, as we look at this as a whole-body procedure, and not just a localized procedure. We want to ensure *all* of your proportions look good.

Your unique genetic makeup may mean that we take fat from certain areas over others so that we can correct any genetic asymmetry. This comes back to the concept of "the frame." You have an existing frame around your buttocks before the surgery, and we are going to base our plan of action around that frame because that is going to determine what we have to leave and what we have to take away in order to achieve your desired outcome. For some women, we may want to take a lot of the fat from their inner and outer thighs, where for others we will want to take more from the stomach and love handles. The BBL procedure isn't the same for a patient who is more barrel shaped or more mid-section heavy as it is for someone carrying most of her excess weight in her legs.

These are some of the things we are looking for while we collect your history and do your physical exam.

We're also going to look for things like loose skin or cellulite. These are things that may or may not change during the procedure, and we want to make sure that you go in with accurate expectations. Patients commonly believe that when we do liposuction and transfer fat to the buttocks, the cellulite is going to magically disappear. Unfortunately, that's not normally the case. It may mask it or decrease the indentations in certain areas, but in general, cellulite is a genetic issue and isn't necessarily going to be affected or improved by liposuction.

After getting your family and personal medical history and completing the physical exam, we will do a thorough assessment to determine whether you are a good match for the procedure and, if so, to get a good idea of what we're starting with and where you want to go. We are taking a good look at the canvas we are starting with, which helps us to create the best plan for your transformation and to set realistic expectations for you.

Once we determine that you meet the necessary physical requirements for the BBL and assess both the starting line and the finish line, then we will discuss with you the exact details of your procedure. This is a little different for every patient. The plan answers questions such as:

- What kind of liposuction are we going to do?

- What parts of the body are we going to take fat from?
- What are the proportions we're aiming for?
- What is the frame we're starting with?
- Where exactly are we transferring the fat to?
- What will be the final shape and measurements we're going for?

This is as much a conversation between a surgeon and his patient as it is an artist and his muse. We are not just focusing on the technical ins and outs of the procedure, but also tapping in to your most intimate desires and hopes for the outcome.

## The Photo

Part of the physical exam in cosmetic surgery is the photo. When you go to your general physician, most of the physical exam is listening to your heart, listening to the lungs, etc. In cosmetic surgery, however, the photo is one of the most important parts of the physical exam because we have to document what we are starting with—the canvas. This is the first step in creating the plan to get where we want to go and setting realistic expectations in the process.

You'd be surprised by how many people forget what they looked like prior to the surgery. I recently had a BBL patient come into my office who had gotten the procedure done a year before. She's a petite woman—probably 5-foot-4-inches, and weighs about 130 pounds. She comes in and says, "I don't notice a difference."

I listen to her concerns, then say, "OK, let's take a picture." I always start with this because you can't argue with a picture. Getting an image of the "after" for the sake of comparison helps the patient to recognize the actual results.

So, we take the picture of her current backend—her "after"—and then put it side-by-side with her "before" picture a year earlier. We look at them together and I say, "What do you think now?"

Her face brightens and she laughs, "My butt looks amazing!"

That's the power of the photograph. She went from, "I don't see a difference," to "I love my butt, it looks amazing" in a matter of seconds.

It's common for people to get so used to what they have that they forget what it was like before the surgery. Their new butt fits their body so naturally that they literally don't remember what they started with. (Perhaps they don't *want* to remember!) This is why photography is a really important part of your physical exam.

## Weight

Because the BBL is a transfer of fat to the buttocks, we first have to make sure there is fat to be transferred. You need to have a little excess fat somewhere on your body, and it's especially helpful if you have it in your midsection. When we do our exam, we're looking for extra fat in the abdomen, flanks, arms, and inner or outer thighs. An average BBL transfers about half a liter to a liter, or 500 to 1000 ccs to each butt cheek. That's the equivalent of a total of one to two liters of excess fat for the entire procedure. So, imagine a two-liter bottle of soda in your mind. That's the amount of fat we need to make the transfer happen. In some cases, when I am trying to make a dramatic change in buttock size, I may use up to 1500 ccs of fat per butt cheek.

The best candidate for this procedure is someone who is a normal size or even slightly overweight, which typically falls within the Body Mass Index (BMI) range of twenty to thirty-two. That's the happy zone because that gives us enough fat to work with, but you're still a healthy individual with little risk under anesthesia. In addition, people who are slightly overweight will have more choices in the shape of the buttocks that they want. They can go small, medium, or large; whereas a normal-weight person may only be able to choose between a small or medium-sized change.

Take a look at this diagram for a great visual on what we're looking for in terms of the ideal BBL body type:

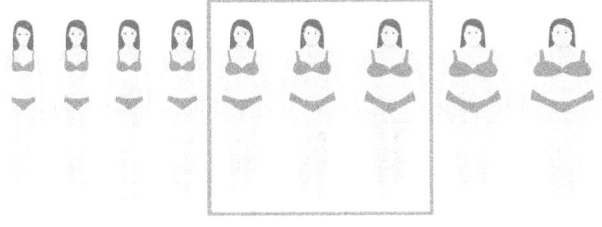

On the left side of the spectrum, we have body types that are too thin for this procedure. If you're really thin, you may not have an extra two liters of fat in your entire body, much less in one or two specific areas. However, this is one of those fluid parameters we discussed earlier. We can talk about you temporarily gaining some weight specifically for this procedure. Or, if that's really just not an option for you, then we can discuss some of the alternative procedures to the BBL that we can use to augment the size and shape of your back end. These alternatives include options like implants or injectable fillers—all of which we will discuss in detail in the next chapter, *Chapter Five: Alternatives to the Brazilian Butt Lift*.

On the opposite end of the spectrum, on the right side, we have the body types that are too overweight for us to safely recommend the procedure. This is also based on your or BMI.

The following table shows the general BMI ranges:[1]

| BMI Ranges | | |
|---|---|---|
| | From | To |
| Low | 0 | 18.5 |
| Normal | 18.5 | 25 |
| Overweight | 25 | 30 |
| Obese (Level 1) | 30 | 35 |
| Obese (Level 2) | 35 | 40 |
| Obese (Level 3) | 40 | 40+ |

Generally, cosmetic surgeons prefer not to do a BBL procedure on BMIs over thirty-two, plus or minus a few points. When you get into that category, you're considered a high-risk patient. You would possibly be denied the procedure, or you would be required to go through additional medical clearances with your primary care physician to ensure that you're healthy enough to undergo the procedure. Of course, again, this is one of those fluid parameters because there is always the option for you to lose weight, at least in the short term, in order to bring your BMI down into a safer range for the procedure.

## How to Calculate Your BMI

You can calculate your own BMI using one of the following formulas, depending on whether you're using the metric system (kilograms and meters for your weight and height) or the English system (pounds and inches for your weight and height:

### Metric BMI Calculation

$$\text{BMI} = \frac{\text{Weight (kg)}}{\text{Height (m)}^2}$$

## English BMI Calculation

$$\text{BMI} = \frac{\text{Weight (lb)}}{\text{Height (in)}^2} \times 703$$

So, let's say you weigh 150 pounds and you are 64 inches (five feet four inches) tall. You would calculate your BMI using the following formula:

$$\text{BMI} = \frac{150}{64^2} \times 703$$

$$\text{BMI} = 25.7$$

This calculation shows that your BMI would be 25.7, which would put you within the ideal range for the BBL procedure.

Once we've qualified you for the procedure based on your health, weight, and body type, we then need to set realistic expectations. If you're a normal-weight person, the amount of fat we can shift to the buttocks is limited, meaning there's not going to be a dramatic increase in the shape and size of the buttocks. As long as you understand that, we can proceed. However, this doesn't mean the procedure won't be a success. If you have a smaller frame, then a smaller augmentation may look the best proportionally to the rest of your body anyway.

## Realistic Expectations

Realistic expectations are a huge part of being an ideal candidate. We begin our assessment by giving you this form to fill out.

1. Please check and initial which body type you think you are:

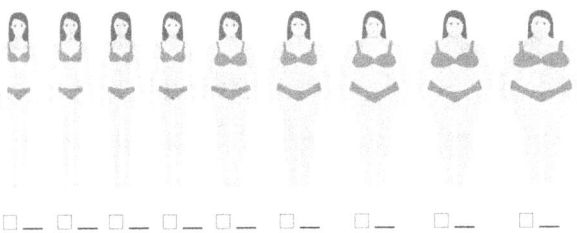

2. Plastic surgery can make vast improvements on your body, but it does have its limits. Please check and initial which body type you would reasonably expect to have after surgery:

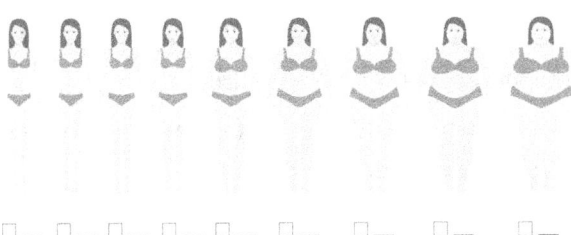

This is a diagram that allows you to assess yourself as you are right now, and also to show us what your expectations are for the BBL procedure. Basically, you're showing us your perspective of your "before," and letting us know your expectations for your "after." This gives us a sense of whether or not we need to spend more time setting realistic expectations so that we can make sure we are on the same page.

For instance, let's say you relate most closely to the body type on the far-right of the diagram—the heaviest one—and so you check that off as your "before." On the second row, you are asked to circle the look you feel you can reasonably expect after your surgery. If you check off the far-left body type on the diagram—the thinnest one possible—then we probably need to have another conversation because that is just not realistic. Not even liposuction can achieve such a drastic change.

The other thing this diagram shows is whether your view of your "before" is already skewed. In addition to setting realistic expectations, we also need to screen for any underlying psychological disorders that can inhibit the way you see yourself. An ideal candidate is going to be in good mental health, too.

One of the most common body disorders we're screening for is called Body Dysmorphic Disorder, which is a disorder that causes you to grossly underestimate or overestimate your size. For example, let's say a woman comes in who is 6-foot tall, weighs ninety pounds, and wants liposuction because she feels overweight. When she looks in the mirror, she actually sees a fat person looking back at her, even though she is extremely thin. We can't operate on patients who have these disorders because no matter what you do to them, they will never see themselves as anybody but the distorted image they have in their minds. Let's say we did perform liposuction on the 6-foot woman in our example. Because she has body dysmorphic disorder, she is likely to come back after the surgery and complain that she is still fat! Surgery will not solve anything and will only make things worse for her.

Cosmetic surgery can attract patients who have these kinds of disorders or who are really unhappy with themselves for other reasons. It's really important for us to make sure we match the right patients with the right procedures. We need to make sure that you are in your right frame of mind and ready for the procedure.

We take all of these steps because in order to have happy patients, it's important that we take the time to make sure that they're the right patients for this procedure. It's just as much about matching the right patient with the right procedure as it is ensuring that we aren't allowing the wrong patient to have the wrong procedure.

When I first started my practice many years ago, I wanted to take on every patient that walked through my door. But after many years of experience and many gray hairs, I have come to realize that some patients just have unrealistic expectations, while others will never be pleased. No matter how hard I work or how hard I try, I don't have any power over their ability to be pleased with the outcome because there is something going on inside of them that is determining their experiences. Whether it's a personal struggle at the time, a mood disorder, or a generally negative disposition—sometimes there is just something going on inside that is going to keep these patients from being satisfied with any work that is done, even if the results are great by any other standard. Before approving you for surgery, we want to make sure that you are doing this for the right reasons. It's important that you are doing this for yourself, not for anyone else, and that you have realistic expectations of what can be achieved with this procedure. Our goal as surgeons is to make you happy. So, we choose our patients wisely—for your sake and for ours.

---

[1] See https://medlineplus.gov/ency/patientinstructions/000348.htm

# CHAPTER FIVE
# *Alternatives to the Brazilian Butt Lift*

Now, I want to discuss with you some of the alternatives to the Brazilian Butt Lift for those instances in which the BBL is not an option. For example, a woman who is very thin and wants a very large change in the appearance of her butt will have to look at alternatives because there just simply isn't going to be enough fat on her body to do a transfer.

However, before I give an overview of the alternatives, I need to stress how strongly I suggest the BBL as your go-to procedure for your augmentation, as long as your unique body type will allow for it. The biggest reason for this is that it is the most natural way to enhance the size of your buttocks because we are using materials that are naturally found in your body. We aren't introducing anything foreign into your body's ecosystem, which makes everything go so much more smoothly and decreases the risk of future complications. There is no risk of your body rejecting the procedure, less risk of infection, and the augmentation will make a more natural transition with your body as you age.

If the BBL is not an option for you, some of the alternatives include:

- Buttock Implants
- Collagen stimulating injections or fillers
- Skin tightening lasers

## Implants

Implants are the generally accepted Plan B. For this procedure, we surgically place a solid silicone implant just above or inside the gluteal muscle on each side. We insert the implant through an incision in the crease of the buttocks, or "butt crack". Once it's in place, the buttocks looks fuller and more round. One benefit of having an implant is that you have a lot of control over the size of your augmentation. The size and shape of the implant is not dependent on the amount of fat you are currently carrying elsewhere. (Of course, your ideal will still be based on your unique body type and proportions.)

However, getting implants is only a semi-permanent procedure, as they may need to be replaced in future. In addition, there are several risks associated with implants, which is why the go-to procedure will always be the BBL for qualified patients.

**These risks include:**

- Infection
- Malposition of the implant
- Pain after surgery
- Capsular contracture

## Infection

The biggest concern with getting implants is the possibility of infection. The incision for the implant is made inside the butt crack, which is uncomfortably close to your "back door," which is teaming with bacteria. It can be a challenge to keep the incision adequately cleaned and protected during the healing process. There are studies that show that almost one third of butt implant patients must eventually have the implant removed because of infection or a seroma—a large, painful pocket of fluid that forms around the implant.[1]

## Capsular Contracture

One of the biggest risks for an implant is that it's a foreign object to the body. Since the implant is manmade, it is not as thoroughly assimilated into your body as your own fat. That means it will always be a foreign object resting in the buttocks. Whenever there is an implant or foreign substance in the body, the body creates a shell around it called a capsule. These capsules hold the implant in place. Ideally, this layer of tissue stays soft and supple, but sometimes it tightens and hardens over time, which compacts the object and makes it feel hard. This is called capsular contracture. If this happens, you are no longer going to be sitting on soft, squishy implants. You will be sitting on rocks. Ouch!

## Malposition of the Implant

Capsules can become wide or loose, which can sometimes cause the implant to move. In 2014, there were rumors and pictures reporting that celebrity Blac Chyna suffered an implant mishap when one of her implants flipped upside down. Although it is uncommon, this can happen. In addition, getting implants is only a semi-permanent procedure, as they may need to be replaced several years later.

## Pain After Surgery

There is significantly more pain during recovery after getting implants because the surgeon needs to stretch and pull the gluteus muscles in order to get the placement just right. This makes the area very sore, and any movement that requires the butt muscles is very painful (you use them more than you think!).

## Collagen Stimulating Injections or Filler Injections

The next option available is having collagen injections, which are comprised of poly-L-lactic acid. It is injected just below the skin and is intended for use in people with healthy immune systems as a one-time treatment regimen of up to four injection sessions that are scheduled about one month apart. Poly-L-lactic acid helps stimulate your skin's own natural collagen production to help restore its inner structure and increase volume that has been lost to aging. However, the change is subtle and takes place over time, gradually thickening the tissue up to four times thicker, which is the main source of the enhancement. The final results will be seen after several months and will last two to three years.

Some of the main drawbacks of this option are that it is not a permanent or dramatic change, and that it is very costly with the promise of only minimal to moderate results. However, this BBL alternative is still popular because it is a non-surgical procedure—usually taking only about thirty minutes—there is no need for anesthesia, and there is essentially no downtime afterwards. You can go back to work or about your normal routine immediately.

## Beware of Black Market Butt Enhancements

Unfortunately, some women look to the black market for injections in order to save a few bucks. In July 2017, the *New York Post* reported the death of a 31-year-old mother who died after getting a black-market injection procedure done to increase the size of her butt. Twelve days after the illegal injections, she called 911 because she was experiencing chest pains and dizziness. She was later pronounced brain dead and taken off of life support.[2]

In 2014, Apryl Brown was working as a hair stylist when one of her clients offered to give her injections that would increase the size of her backside. Brown jumped at the promise of a bigger buttocks at a fraction of the price. After receiving her second of four scheduled injections, however, she developed a severe staph infection, and the doctors had to amputate her hands, feet, and flesh from her butt and hips in order to save her life. An investigation showed that she had been injected with bathroom caulk. Today, she works to bring awareness to the risks associated with these black-market cosmetic procedures.[3]

These black-market trends are increasing in popularity because women are not aware of the dangers associated with these procedures. More and more, there are reports of so-called "Pumping Parties." People go to these parties for the sole purpose of increasing the size of their breasts or butts by allowing an unlicensed physician to pump illegal and outlandish materials into the desired area. These materials include but are not limited to substances such as concrete, tire filler, and super glue.

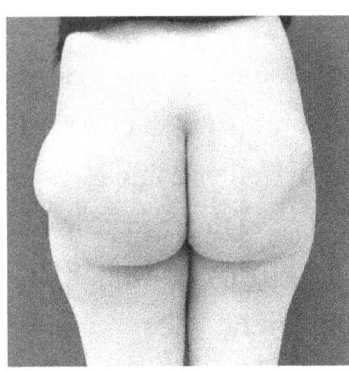

*This is an example of a BBL complication after injection of a non-FDA approved filler. (Image courtesy of Dr. Tarick Smiley)*

The most common illegal filler being used is industrial or commercial-grade silicone. People hear the word "silicone" and don't realize there is a spectrum of grades and qualities. The silicone used in implants is a very different material than the silicone fillers being illegally used on the black market. Commercial-grade silicone is not safe for the human body, nor was it ever designed to be. It is detrimental to body tissues. In addition, it comes in a "loose" form, which is very different than the solid implants used in approved surgical procedures. When a loose substance is injected into the bum, it is not necessarily going to stay in the bum. It is just as likely to travel to other areas in the body. Aside from creating an obvious issue with the shape of the buttocks, this will also lead to other health risks as the body works to fight against this intruder. Commercial grade Silicone is not sterile and can cause life-threatening infections.

Even if the procedure doesn't kill or permanently maim you, there are other complications that you will likely face such as the site becoming dark and leathery, or the weight of the injections causing excessive sagging and deforming the shape of the butt.

It's important that you recognize the dangers that these illegal procedures pose. They simply are not worth the risk to your body or to your life. In the United States, there are only twenty-one FDA approved dermal fillers—none of which are approved for self-injection or by anyone other than a licensed practitioner. Stepping outside the protective care of a licensed physician is a risky, and potentially lethal, endeavor that should be avoided at all costs.

## Skin Tightening Lasers

Another option for improving the appearance of your buttocks is the use of skin tightening lasers and technology. This methodology is exactly what it sounds like. It uses skin tightening lasers and technologies to tighten the buttocks skin and stimulate collagen production to create a fuller, rounder and more lifted appearance.

As women age, they produce less estrogen and collagen, and their skin loses elasticity. This technology combats that with non-invasive procedures that offer noticeable results that typically last a few years. This technique does not allow you to modify the natural shape of your back end, but it does help to restore it back to its more youthful, shapely form. This improvement takes time, though, because it relies heavily on the gradual increase in collagen. It may take anywhere from three to six months before you see your final results.

Popular methodologies that employ this technology are radio frequency, ultrasound heat, and infrared treatments. There is some variance between each of these treatments, but the overall goals and procedures are similar, and none of them require much, if any, downtime.

## Other Options

In addition, you can try some at-home avenues, such as:

- Topical creams: There are creams that have been formulated to plump up your fat cells over time, which creates a small enhancement to the size of your butt.
- Supplements: Some supplements claim they can steer your body to store more fat on your hips and butt. However, it's important to note that most of these claims have not been verified by any clinical studies to prove their efficacy.

- Exercise: There are specific exercises you can do to enlarge your gluteal muscles and give your backend a more natural lift (i.e. squats and lunges). However, these results are gradual and are dependent on your consistent and long-term effort.
- Padded underwear: This is a quick way to augment the appearance of your bum without actually augmenting it.

There are many things to consider when you're choosing which option is going to be the best fit with your long-term goals and desires. While we definitely recognize the BBL to be the safest and most attractive procedure, we also know that it is not always an option for all of our patients.

---

[1] See http://www.theplasticsurgerychannel.com/2017/04/19/butt-implant-complications/

[2] "Woman killed by botched butt injection," 31 July 2017; https://nypost.com/2017/07/31/woman-killed-by-botched-butt-injection/.

[3] "DIY Plastic Surgery Leads to Horrific Injuries," 2 July 2014; https://www.cnn.com/2014/07/01/health/diy-plastic-surgery/index.html.

# CHAPTER SIX
## *Preparing for Your Surgery*

Serena comes in the day of her Brazilian Butt Lift procedure, and I can tell she is nervous. This is normal. After all, this *is* surgery. As we go through the pre-op checklist, she is smiling, but her tremble does not go unnoticed. Just before we begin, I reach for her hand.

"Serena, we're going to take good care of you. I promise." I smile warmly. "Now, what is your most favorite place in all the world? I want you to tell me what it is and get that picture in your mind."

She thinks a moment then smiles. "Maui.

Definitely Maui." Her hand is still in mine, and I can feel her relax a little bit.

"Yes, that's a beautiful place. What do you love most about it?"

"The beaches."

"The beaches. OK. I want you to think about those beaches. Think about the blue water, the way it feels to have that tropical breeze blowing across your body, and the warmth of the sunshine. Maybe you're sipping on your favorite mixed drink and holding hands with someone you love. Do you have that picture in your mind?"

She nods.

"OK, Serena, you're going to go to sleep now, and I want you to stay right there on that beach for me until we're done. Do you think you can do that for me?"

Her smile is genuine as she nods again, and I notice she's no longer trembling.

I give her hand a small squeeze, and now it's time to begin.

Once your BBL has been scheduled, there are going to be a lot of things to do, and a lot of things to feel. Before I get into the dry details of the "dos and don'ts" beforehand, I first want to talk with you about the things that you will be feeling. This is extremely important.

Throughout the process of deciding to do your surgery, having it done, recovering, and then moving on with your life afterward, you're going to be on a bit of an emotional roller coaster, and I want you to be prepared for that. First and foremost, I want you to know that this roller coaster is completely normal.

The emotional stages patients experience after recovery affects each person differently. The stages I talk about below are just a basic outline and the general expectation, but your personal happiness curve may follow a different path. For instance, the most common reaction is to be depressed on the third or fourth day. However, some patients say, "Well, not me. I didn't feel depressed." But three weeks later, they may start crying while driving to work. Whatever your curve looks like, be patient with yourself and remember that we are just a phone call or a short drive away when you need additional support.

PREPARING FOR YOUR SURGERY

## The Happiness Curve

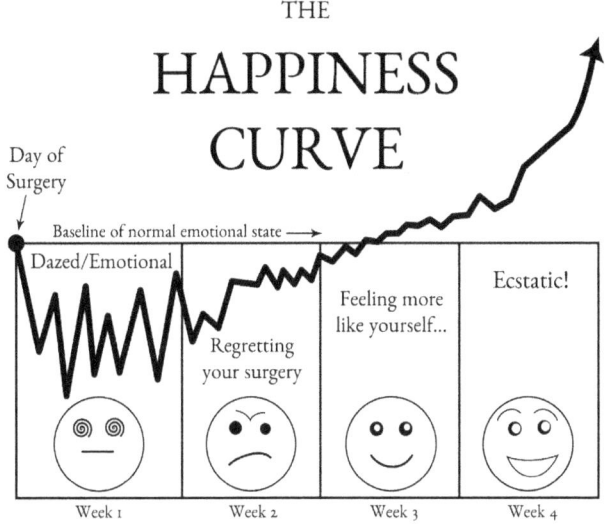

Starting out, you will feel pretty excited about the changes that are coming. However, as it gets closer, you will start to feel nervous and possibly even afraid about the procedure itself. I see this when you come in. And I understand. If you're a Type A personality like me, and you want to be in control of the details of your life, anesthesia can be a terrifying experience because it leaves you very vulnerable.

Right before you fall asleep, I will hold your hand, too, and look you right in the eyes as I assure you that we are going to take great care of you. I promise you we will. Then, I will have you imagine the happiest place in the world for you and really get that picture in your mind before we start the anesthesia. You can dream under anesthesia, so if I can get you to visualize your happiest place before you fall asleep, it's my hope that is what you will dream about, too. If nothing else, it will be the last thing you think about before you fall asleep, and the first thing you think about when you wake up. That is significantly better than whatever fears and worries may be swirling around in your mind beforehand.

Right after the surgery, you will feel a bit like a zombie for the first day or two as the anesthesia wears off and as you deal with the fog from the pain medication. You'll mostly want to sleep. But after that, you're going to move into what I call "the antsy" stage and you will be feeling some intense emotion in that first week. You're going to be in pain, and your life will be on hold for a short period of time as you heal. You're going to have a lot of time to think, and you will most likely be asking yourself, "What have I done?" You may be angry at yourself for doing this, or even with me for doing it to you! You may even regret going through the procedure. These are all normal feelings during the first week.

After that, you will move into what I call "the weirdo" stage of the happiness curve. This is going to be about week two after the surgery. You're still going to be a little swollen, and you're going to be looking at your butt and complaining that it isn't right—that's not what you wanted it to look like. This realization is going to make you feel scared. During our post-surgery visits, I will assure you that this is normal and that it's still in the process of changing. Then, your fear will be replaced with impatience as you say, "I just want it to be a month from now already!"

As you move into the third and fourth week of recovery, you will stop complaining as you start getting back to your normal routine. Then, suddenly, you will be surprised by your first compliment. Other people will begin commenting on your improved appearance, and you will begin to notice how amazing you look.

However, something may begin to eat at you, and your mind might also play tricks on you. You may not put your finger on it right away. But in a quiet moment one night, it will occur to you that you resent the attention. Why didn't you have that kind of attention before? What does this say about you? Or, about the people who are admiring you now?

Listen. I understand your concerns, and why these questions are important to you. But what it comes down to is that you decided to get the procedure in order to boost your confidence and give you an edge. This new attention is proof that it was a success. You are not someone else now that you have made an improvement to your appearance. You are simply *more you*.

As you grow into this new perspective of your new life, there will be a moment when you find yourself miraculously immersed in joy. You will suddenly find yourself at the top of that happiness curve—in love with your new look, the new attention, and the way it feels to be so fully in your own skin. You will also see how strong you are—that you can do hard things with courage and with grace. Suddenly, you will see what I see in you—that you are a person of courage who can demand great deeds from yourself. And you will.

## Getting Ready for Surgery

As we get closer to the surgery, it's time to get into the pre-operative instructions. Preparation begins up to four weeks prior to your surgery and continues up until the procedure itself. If you require medical clearance from your regular physician for any reason—whether it's age, weight, or health-related—we require that you obtain clearance at least two weeks prior to your surgery, so it's important to schedule those appointments (e.g. EKG, blood work, mammogram) right away to give you time to navigate wait times.

It's important to be thorough in your preparation beforehand, keeping in mind that our instructions are meant to ensure your overall safety, a smooth procedure, and a fast recovery period.

## Four Weeks Prior to Surgery

There is to be absolutely *no* smoking or nicotine use for the month before *and* after your surgery. Zero! This is because nicotine use can reduce your blood flow, which results in an overall decrease in the oxygenation of your blood and body. Specifically, this means that the cut edges of your incisions are not going to have the oxygen and nutrients they need to heal properly. Poor healing can lead to undesirable scars or even skin breakdown during recovery.

## Two Weeks Prior to Surgery

Two weeks prior, you need to avoid taking any blood-thinning medications or supplements because these will inhibit blood clotting and blood coagulation during the procedure. Blood thinners include medications and supplements such as aspirin, ibuprofen, Aleve, herbs such as St. John's wart, various brands of diet pills, or high doses of vitamin E or fish oils. (See the detailed list of medications to avoid in the Appendix.) It's best to just discontinue using supplements and vitamins altogether at this point—with the exception of those mentioned below—because it is hard to know if there are any blood-thinning medications or ingredients in them. You can resume taking them a week after the procedure.

Tylenol or extra-strength Tylenol is fine to

use up to the day of the procedure, as that's the only pain reliever that doesn't have a blood-thinning effect. We also recommend that you start taking specific supplements such as Arnica Montana and Bromelain at this point, and continue taking them throughout your recovery period, in order to promote your optimum health before and after the procedure, as these will help reduce bruising and swelling after surgery.

## Overview

- No aspirin or medicines that contain aspirin* because it interferes with normal blood clotting.
- No ibuprofen or medicines that contain ibuprofen* because it interferes with blood clotting.
- Discontinue all herbal medications* because many have side effects that could complicate a surgical procedure by inhibiting blood clotting, affecting blood pressure, or interfering with anesthetics.
- Discontinue all diet pills—whether prescription, over-the-counter, or herbal—as many

will interfere with anesthesia and can cause cardiovascular concerns.

- No mega doses of Vitamin E, although a multiple vitamin that contains Vitamin E is fine to take up to one week prior and you can resume one week after surgery.
- Absolutely no smoking because nicotine reduces blood flow to the skin and can cause significant complications during healing. In some states, Marijuana use is legal, and some surgeons may allow or recommend edible versions of marijuana (or its derivatives THC or CBD) to be used for post-operative pain control. However, smoking marijuana is still harmful to the healing process.
- Start taking the recommended supplements each day and continue taking this through your recovery. The healthier you are, the quicker your recovery will be.

\* See *Medications to Avoid* in the Appendix

## One Week Prior to Surgery

As you get closer to the surgery date—about a week out—reduce the use of short-term blood thinners—specifically alcohol. Alcohol is a blood thinner and also interferes with anesthesia so avoid use until at least one week after the surgery. This would include the use of cough and cold medications.

## Your Caregiver

Now is also the time to make arrangements for someone to drive you to and from the procedure, as well as someone who can spend the first twenty-four hours with you after. The key here is to choose someone who's *really* going to take care of you—both physically and emotionally. You don't want to go home to someone whose first comment to you is going to be, "What the heck did you do this for?" Trust me—you're going to be wondering that enough yourself those first few days. Instead, you need someone who will be compassionate and understanding, and who will happily hold your hand through those rough days as they reassure you that everything is going to be OK. You're going to need that kind of warmth and support.

## Overview

- Do not take or drink any alcohol or drugs beginning one week prior to your surgery and until at least one week after your surgery, as these can interfere with anesthesia and affect blood clotting.
- Do not take any cough or cold medications without permission.
- Begin using a germ-inhibiting soap for bathing, such as Dial, Safeguard, or Lever (as long as your skin can tolerate it).
- Report any signs of cold, infection, boils, or pustules appearing before surgery.
- Make arrangements for a responsible adult to drive you to and from the facility on the day of your surgery. You will not be allowed to leave on your own.
- Make arrangements for a responsible individual to spend the first twenty-four hours with you. You cannot be left alone.

## Night Prior to and Morning of Surgery

Be sure to bathe or shower the night before the procedure using anti-bacterial soap (if your skin will allow for it), and again the morning of. It's also recommended that you shave any underarm or pubic hairs because these can harbor bacteria. Shaving tends to make the skin a little cleaner and reduces the risk of infection because it prevents hairs getting caught in sutures and stitches.

Make sure not to apply any sprays, lotions, gels, perfumes, or powders—anything that sticks to the skin or that acts like a barrier to the skin. We prep the site beforehand with things like iodine and other powerful antibacterial agents, but if there are creams or lotions on the skin they may interfere with the ability of these surgical cleansers to clean the skin properly.

Do not eat or drink anything after midnight the night before because your stomach has to be empty when you go under anesthesia. Anytime you're having either twilight sedation or general anesthesia, you're not allowed to eat or drink after midnight the day before due to the risk of aspirating. Stomach acid and/or food can travel up the stomach and into the lungs, which creates a severe risk for pneumonia. So, it's really crucial that you don't eat or drink *anything*—no gum, candy, mints, coffee—not even water. (You can brush your teeth, but be careful not to swallow any water.) All of these can cause risks while you're under anesthesia and pose a risk for aspiration.

Don't wear contact lenses during your surgery because you won't have full control of your eyes opening and closing during the procedure. It's better to come with your regular glasses on.

Wear loose, comfortable clothing. This is very important because you will be sore afterwards and will likely also be swollen. You want to be sure to wear something you can easily put on and take off without having to go over your head, such as button-down tops and sweat pants.

It's always a good idea not to bring anything valuable—no jewelry, no expensive watches, or anything like that. It's best to leave these kinds of things at home. In addition to limiting the possibility of loss, the metal can sometimes interfere with anesthesia and certain machines that we use during surgery.

Again, it's critical that you've made arrangements for someone to drive you to and from your surgery. These procedures are done under anesthesia, so you are prohibited from driving yourself. We require an emergency contact and encourage you to bring a friend or family member who can take you home after your surgery. An average procedure lasts anywhere between two and three hours, depending on how many areas of liposuction we're doing and how much fat is being transferred during the BBL.

You are also required to have someone who will be able to stay with you the first twenty-four hours after your surgery. If you are not recovering at home, it is very important that we have the number where you will be staying so that we can check in on you and see how you're doing.

## Overview

- Do not eat or drink anything (not even water) after midnight the night before your surgery and until after the surgery. Do not sneak anything, as this may endanger you.

- Clear any regular medications you're taking with your surgeon beforehand.
- Take a thorough shower with germ-inhibiting soap the night before and the morning of surgery.
- Be sure to shampoo or shave your underarm and pubic hair the morning of surgery. This is to decrease the bacteria on the skin, which will thereby decrease the risk of infection.
- Do not apply any of the following to your skin, hair, or face the morning of surgery: makeup, cream, lotion, hair gel, body spray, perfume, powder, or deodorant. Using any of these products will add bacteria to the skin and increase the risk of infection.
- You may brush your teeth the morning of surgery, but do not drink anything.
- Do not wear contacts to surgery. If you bring glasses, bring your eyeglass case.
- Wear comfortable, loose-fitting clothes that do not have to be put on over your head. The best things to wear home are a loose button-up top and loose pull-on pants. You will also want flat shoes that are easy to slip on.

- Do not bring any valuables or wear any jewelry (no rings, earrings, chains, toe rings, other metal piercings, or watches). We will need to tape wedding rings if worn.
- You must have another adult drive you to and from surgery. Please note that a cab or bus driver will not be allowed to take you home after surgery. On arrival, be sure we know your drivers' names, phone numbers, and how we will be able to reach them.

Again, it's important to keep in mind that these instructions are for *your* benefit and safety. Please be thorough in your preparation, and be sure to speak up if you have any concerns or questions beforehand. Our team is always focused on providing the highest customer service possible. Following these guidelines down to the very last detail helps us help you have a safe, smooth procedure, and a fast recovery.

# CHAPTER SEVEN
## *Post-Op and Recovery*

After your BBL procedure has been done, your recovery will come in phases. Please be sure to follow these instructions very carefully, as this will ensure the best outcome and results from your procedure as well as the fastest and most comfortable recovery period possible. Some patients are tempted to skip some of these steps because they are anxious to jump back into their normal routines or because the urge to smoke again is so strong. However, they quickly discover that this is a mistake.

I have performed this procedure many times in my career, and I can assure you that no one is exempt from these guidelines. Your life can wait for you. Taking the necessary time to recover, and following these instructions with precision, will ensure that you return to your normal routine as your best self as quickly as possible.

The first four weeks after the procedure are the most important—both physically and emotionally—in your recovery period. You can expect a measure of soreness and discomfort during this time, and you will need to take the precautions detailed below in order to avoid damaging your augmentation. This is one reason why you will be asked to wear a compression garment during recovery. It will help manage the swelling immediately after the procedure, while also promoting healthy drainage. The compression garment will not be so tight as to stress the transplanted cells, but will be snug enough to do its job after your surgery.

**Note:** Some surgeons do not require compression garments at all.

## Days One and Two

As previously mentioned, for the first couple days after your surgery, you're going to be recovering from the anesthesia and coping with the fog of the pain medication. You're going to be very dependent on the person you have chosen to take care of you. Again, I can't stress enough the importance of carefully choosing your caregiver and ensuring it's someone up to the emotional and physical task of helping you during this very vulnerable period of time.

**Here's an overview of the additional things you need to be aware of and prepare for during this stage of recovery:**

- You must have an adult drive you home from our office after surgery. You will not be allowed to drive yourself or use public transportation.
- After surgery, you must have a responsible adult stay with you for a minimum of twenty-four hours, which begins when you are discharged. You cannot be left alone. This is important because of the risk of falling, losing your concept of time, or possibly overmedicating yourself.
- The effects of anesthesia can persist for twenty-four hours. You must exercise extreme caution before engaging in any activity that could be harmful to yourself or others.

- It is very important to keep well hydrated, as drinking fluids will help rid your body of the drugs used in surgery. Using straws is helpful because people tend to drink more fluids that way. Drink at least eight ounces of fluid every one to two hours, avoiding caffeinated beverages. Staying hydrated can also help prevent your blood pressure from dropping too low, which is common after surgery.
- Avoid spicy, fatty, fried, or salty foods the first forty-eight hours. Your first meal after surgery should be bland (soup, toast, bananas, Jell-O, crackers, etc.). If that's tolerated, then you can progress back to your regular diet.
- Avoid the use of alcoholic beverages for the first seven days (it dilates blood vessels and can cause unwanted bleeding) and as long as pain medications are being used (this is a very dangerous combination). Alcohol is also a blood thinner, which can also cause postoperative bleeding.
- Take only medications that have been prescribed by your surgeon for your postoperative care, and take them according to the

instructions on the bottle. Your pain medication may make you feel "spacey," so it's best to have another adult help to administer these to avoid accidental overdose.

- If you experience any generalized itching, rash, wheezing, or tightness in the throat, stop taking all medications and call the office immediately, as this may be a sign of a drug allergy.
- The greatest discomfort is usually during the first forty-eight hours, which should be helped by the pain medications. Thereafter, you will find that you require less pain medication. Call your doctor if you experience severe pain that is not helped by pain medications. It is not unusual to not need pain medication the first twelve hours after surgery due to the numbing effect of the tumescent anesthesia that most surgeons use during a BBL procedure.
- Keep all of your dressings on, clean, and dry. Do not remove them until instructed to do so. There may be some bloody drainage on the dressings. If you have excessive bleeding or the bandages are too tight, call the office immediately.

- It is important to have a bowel movement within a few days of your surgery. Take over-the-counter laxatives if necessary, such as psyllium, docusate, and magnesium citrate.
- Maintain minimal activity for the first forty-eight hours. No house cleaning, furniture rearranging, etc. Relax, be pampered, and let your body heal. The less energy you use on doing things, the more energy your body can expend on healing.
- You are requested to remain within a reasonable traveling distance of the office for approximately the first ten days.
- You may resume showering after your post-op evaluation a few days after surgery (assuming all goes well). No baths should be taken for two weeks. However, gentle sponge baths during the first few days are usually ok.
- Absolutely no smoking for the first four weeks post-operatively. Any cheating will delay healing and may lead to severe complications. Smoking inhibits oxygen from being delivered to the healing areas of your body.

- You may drive two to three days after anesthesia, once you are off the pain pills, and when you experience no pain with this activity (you need to be able to react quickly). When you begin to drive, make sure you are sitting on a soft Boppy pillow to protect your BBL results. Sitting on hard surfaces can crush or put excessive pressure on the newly transferred fat cells.

## Weeks One and Two

After the first couple of days after your surgery, you're going to move into that "antsy" part of the happiness curve. You're going to be sore and possibly a little unhappy. You're going to wonder what you've done, and may be feeling some deep regret over your decision to do this procedure. This is normal. This stage of recovery is an intensely vulnerable period. You are still heavily dependent on your caregiver, and your augmentation isn't going to look like the final product you were hoping for yet.

You are potentially going to have a lot of

private moments in the bathroom while you're looking down at your butt and wondering why you did this to yourself.

My team and I will be there to help you through this stage. We will hold your hand and assure you that your surgery site is still healing and changing, and that it will be beautiful very soon. I promise. Even still, you may just wish you could fast forward through all the discomfort and frustration to that moment *right now*. I understand. Hang in there. It's coming.

**Here's an overview of the additional things you need to be aware of and prepare for during this stage of recovery:**

## Physical Activity

Resume light to normal activity as tolerated. Walking to the bathroom, kitchen, and around the house is recommended, but you must have assistance to do so. It is important to walk to the bathroom—or even take a light walk if you can—in order to get your circulation flowing. This helps minimize the risk of blood clots forming in your calves post-operatively. Every hour while resting, extend your toes as if you were pressing the gas pedal on your car. This will help to promote good circulation.

However, *do not* confuse this with exercise.

Avoid all fat-burning exercises, or any other form of rigorous physical activity during this phase of recovery. That kind of activity will put a lot of strain on your surgery site. Also, avoid any physical activity that puts strain on the area or stretches the skin, such as yoga, stretching exercises, or sexual activity.

Also, there should be no lifting over five pounds for the first two weeks.

## Cleanliness

You may resume showering after your post-op evaluation a few days after surgery (assuming all goes well). *You should not take any baths for two weeks.* When showering, do *not* use hot water, but lukewarm water is OK. Continue using antibacterial soap when washing. This will help minimize the risk of infection.

You can expect your liposuction sites to drain for up to a week after surgery. Your garments can become saturated from the drainage, so be sure to dress the area, and pick your wardrobe accordingly. Keep your dressings clean and dry. If the tape becomes wet or moist, then dry with a hairdryer on the *cool* setting, being sure to hold it at an arm's distance away. Continuously move the hairdryer from side to side; do *not* let it remain in one spot. Do not take off or peel the tape.

If you notice any blisters, redness, or dark areas, call our office immediately.

## Fluids and Diet

It is very important to keep well hydrated. Drink at least eight ounces of fluid every one to two hours for the first ten days, avoiding caffeinated beverages.

Fluids and food are very important components of the healing process. If a full meal is too heavy for you initially, then make sure you are snacking often. Above all, remember that this is not just a butt procedure—it is a whole-body procedure. Be sure to give your *body* the rest and nourishment it needs to recover from your surgery. Eat well-balanced meals, especially in the days immediately following your procedure, and sleep as much as possible. Eating green vegetables or beets rich with iron can help replace the blood that was lost during the procedure. Restoring your iron and B-12 levels can also help bring back your energy levels quickly.

## Smoking

You are *absolutely prohibited* from smoking for the first four weeks after your BBL because this will dramatically affect your body's ability to heal. Smoking has a negative effect on your circulation, and circulation is key to healing. Blood is the lifeforce of your body, so help your body help you: do not smoke. Any cheating could result in significant complications.

## Sleeping

When you're sleeping, do not sleep on your back

under any circumstances. Sleep on your side or stomach, alternating sides every ninety minutes for the first four weeks after recovery. It's important to keep the time intervals even on each side, so you will want to set an alarm to alert you to make the switch during the night. When changing positions, do so slowly. Moving slowly and waiting in between positions will prevent additional dizziness and lightheadedness.

Sleeping on your side can be hard if you're accustomed to sleeping on your back. If that's the position you're used to, you may want to nestle a pillow behind you to help you avoid inadvertently moving into your usual back position while you're sleeping.

## Sitting Down

It's best to avoid sitting down or putting any undue pressure on your BBL during the first four weeks. Not only will this keep you most comfortable (you'll still be a bit sore), but sitting on the injection sites puts pressure on the newly transferred fat cells, which can damage the cells and make them die off faster than you want them to. You should expect 40 percent of the injected fat cells to die off in the first few weeks, which is normal. However, if you put a lot of pressure on the site during recovery, you could end up losing much more than that.

If you have to sit, don't sit down for more than a few minutes at a time, and always use a soft cushion or a Boppy pillow with the opening faced toward the back of your seat. This will cushion the site and help you be more comfortable, but it's still recommended only as a last resort to avoiding sitting all together.

This period of recovery in which you avoid sitting or lying on the procedure site is vital because the body is working to create new blood vessels to feed and heal the area. The more blood vessels you have, the better your circulation. The better your circulation, the better your recovery. The better your recovery, the better the outcome of your BBL.

## Medications

You can resume taking your daily medications unless they contain aspirin, in which case you need to wait one week, as aspirin is a blood thinner, which can affect your recovery.

You will be prescribed pain medications during recovery. Do not consume alcoholic beverages while taking these medications.

**Call your doctor immediately if you experience any of these symptoms:**

- Fever over 101°F
- Excessive redness or swelling, especially if there is more swelling on one side than the other
- Significant increase in drainage and/or odor
- You cannot urinate or you experience pain or pressure in the bladder area at any time.
- You notice any blisters, redness, or dark areas around the liposuction sites.
- You experience severe pain that is not responding to pain medication.
- Your incisions are red or very warm to the touch.

## Week Three

This is when you're going to start getting back into your normal routine. You will likely be cleared to go back to work, which means you're going to be seeing a lot more people. This may be your first public showing of the new you. This is potentially going to bring a lot of emotions with it. Some people may question your decision to make this change, and others may be admiring your new rear end. In either instance, several emotions will probably be stirring inside of you.

Some patients resent the new positive attention. They want to know why they weren't getting the attention they wanted before. They start to wonder what that means about them, or about the people who are admiring them. These questions go deep. I understand. So, this is the best time to remind you that you are not actually a new person. You are still you. You are just a little more you now. The decision to get this procedure was based on a lot of things, and one of them was to boost your self-confidence. Instead of labeling the new attention as something questionable, just use that as your indicator that you have achieved what you set out to do. You are more attractive—both inside and out. Your improved self-confidence makes you glow. Don't second guess yourself.

**At this stage of recovery, you should also note:**

Since you are more than likely to be cleared to return back to work at this stage, it is expected that you will be sitting for a long period of time. Be sure to prop yourself up on your Boppy pillow any time you're sitting down.

Light cardiovascular activities are OK, but don't start running marathons.

Continue to sleep on your side or stomach during week three.

## Weeks Four and Five

At this point in your recovery, you're going to be feeling pretty good physically. You're going to be almost entirely back to your normal routine, and suddenly, there's going to be a day in there that you realize that you look magnificent. Suddenly, you will find yourself at the peak of the happiness curve, immersed in pure joy. You're going to be enjoying the compliments and the attention from others, as well as taking longer looks at yourself as you walk by store windows. This is the sweet spot of recovery.

**Here's an overview of the additional things you need to be aware of and prepare for during this stage of recovery:**

At this point in recovery, you should still be using a pillow any time you're sitting down for longer than a few minutes at a time. However, you're free to step it up a notch with your exercise routine. Nothing too aggressive, but you can pick up the pace when you're walking and use machines like the elliptical. Avoid biking because of the pressure of the seat on your BBL site. Swimming is a great exercise option because it doesn't put any pressure on the site—not even gravity!

In week five, you can start bringing in some weight training exercises. If you are going to exercise, weight training is actually preferred. Avoiding highly aerobic activities that burn a lot of fat will give your transplanted fat cells time and an opportunity to stabilize and "stick."

Continue to sleep on your stomach or side.

## Weeks Six through Eight

At this point, you are relatively free to resume your normal routines in all areas. Your fat cells have had the time they need to stabilize, so you can go back to fat-burning exercises like running, biking, or other rigorous sports. If you're still experiencing any discomfort or soreness, you should come back in for an evaluation.

You can now finally resume sleeping on your back, if that is your preference.

## Additional Precautions During Recovery

- Use sunscreen. All surgeries involve some scarring, which can take up to a year to fade. No matter how small they may be, we still want them to heal as well as they are able. Exposing red scars to the sun can cause permanent discoloration. A good sunscreen (SPF 30 or higher) can help and will protect the surrounding tissues that might not feel a sunburn developing while the nerves are healing. Sunlight can even

reach scars under a swimsuit, so take adequate precautions.
- Do not use a hot tub for four weeks.
- Avoid sports or strenuous activities for four to six weeks as your surgeon gives you clearance during your post-operative visits. This is to avoid any unnecessary complications (bleeding, bruising, swelling).

## Possible Risks of the BBL

It's important to stay in touch with our office, or the office of your surgeon, during your recovery period so that we can monitor your healing. All surgeries come with some risks, and the Brazilian Butt Lift is no different. Some of these possible risks include[1]:

- Anesthesia risks
- Asymmetries
- Bleeding (hematoma)
- Deep vein thrombosis, cardiac, and pulmonary complications
- Fat necrosis, which means that some of the fatty tissue under the skin dies off.

- Fat Embolism, which means some of the fat cells enter the blood stream and block blood flow to the lungs. This is an extremely rare complication that can be avoided with proper surgical technique.
- Fluid accumulation under the skin (seroma)
- Infection
- Numbness or other changes in skin sensation
- Poor wound healing
- Problems with your sutures
- Recurrent looseness of skin
- Serious side effects, such as extreme pain and discomfort during your healing period.
- Skin discoloration and/or prolonged swelling
- Skin loss
- Too much fat being reabsorbed back into your body and away from your buttocks area. This is uncommon but may require a secondary fat transfer in order to achieve your desired results.
- Unfavorable scarring
- Unmet expectations. We do our best to set realistic expectations with you beforehand, but sometimes the outcome is not what you

hoped for. In those instances, you can talk with your surgeon about the best way to address the gap between what you hoped for and what you've achieved.

All of these potential risks will be thoroughly discussed with you prior to your surgery. The best way to avoid these and other complications are to explicitly follow the pre- and post-operative instructions provided.

---

[1] See https://www.plasticsurgery.org/cosmetic-procedures/buttock-enhancement/safety.

## CHAPTER EIGHT
# What Happens to My BBL Over Time?

When you're considering getting the Brazilian Butt Lift, you are probably thinking a lot about how it's going to improve your appearance right now or how it's going to boost your self-confidence at the moment. It's also important to ask questions about the long-term effects of this procedure. Historically, there have been cosmetic surgery trends that didn't serve women for the long haul of their lives. Large breast implants, for instance, may have seemed like a good idea for their immediate effect on a woman's life, but she may have failed to calculate the strain it would put on her body over the course of her lifetime as she was tasked with carrying them around. Perhaps she realized too late that the chronic back pain was not worth the dramatic promotion in cup size.

Fortunately, the BBL is a much more natural procedure. There are almost no physical side effects to this procedure—neither in the short term or the long term. However, there are a few changes you will experience during the life of your BBL. You want to be aware of these in order to have accurate expectations as you move forward.

## The First and Second Change

The first thing you need to be aware of is that there are phases to your augmentation. You will lose 30 to 40 percent of the fat that is transferred to your buttocks within the first few weeks after your surgery. This is normal. This happens while your body is adjusting to the change and working to establish a new blood supply to these cells. Up to 40 percent of those cells die off in the process. That sounds shocking because it's almost half of what we put in. However, that doesn't mean that you are getting less than you bargained for. We compensate for this by over-filling in the first place. After a few weeks, the new blood supply is adequately intact, the cells stabilize, and the shrinkage stops. Over time, the stem cells in your fat will regenerate and replenish some of the size you lose in those first few weeks.

So, you'll have cycles. First you have a shrinkage, then a plateau, and then a little bit of growth again from the stem cells that become fat cells in the area. You should expect to see your final results in about three to six months.

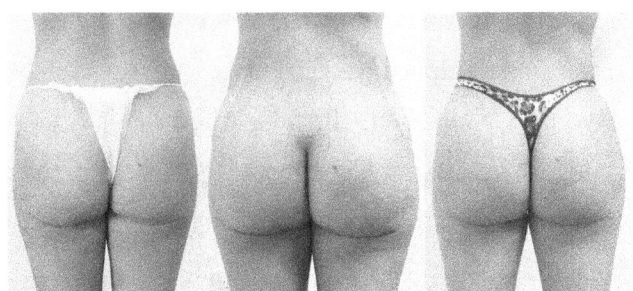

## The Lifetime of the BBL

The Brazilian Butt Lift is a semi-permanent procedure, mostly due to the fact that, by nature, your fat is only semi-permanent. The nature of your fat—the way it is stored, its health, where it is deposited—changes throughout a woman's life. Once the fat graft has stabilized, it will react the same as any other butt. Its shape will still be affected by your weight loss or weight gain, age, and gravity—just as it would be without having the procedure performed. It's recommended that you strive to maintain your normal weight in order to preserve your optimal results.

Over a period of eight to ten years, you may have some loss in volume just from repeated sitting, gaining and losing weight, and the fact that fat cells naturally tend to atrophy and die over time. For example, if you compare a photograph of a woman when she is thirty to when she is fifty—even if she hasn't lost any weight during that time—the pictures will look different. The fifty-year-old face will be thinner, and she will appear to have lost weight, even though she hasn't. This is because our faces become more skeletonized as we get older because the nature of our fat changes. Gravity and loss of elasticity also stretch the skin and fat cells in a downward direction, which can also make the face look thinner and flatter. The same is true for our butts as well. It is natural that as we get older, we lose fat in certain areas of our body—even if we have not lost weight—because fat cells tend to atrophy, or shrink, over time. You can see an exaggeration of this phenomenon in women who are in their eighties and nineties. At that point, you start to see a lot of loose skin because they've lost a lot of their skin's fat layer and elasticity. The National Institute of Health states that all cells experience changes with age. They become less able to divide and multiply.[1]

Many of these changes become more pronounced as women go through menopause, which the NIH says occurs most often between the ages of forty-five and fifty-five. This hormonal shift in your body affects the way that your body stores fat. As your estrogen decreases, you are more prone to have a build up of fat on your abdomen than on your backend. Your collagen production also goes down, which will cause the buttocks to lose some of their firmness and smooth appearance.

This is why the BBL is only considered a semi-permanent augmentation. Even though this is a permanent fat transfer, fat, by nature, is not a permanent thing. I have always told patients, "You can fight mother nature, but she's going to win in the end."

While these changes do take place, there's no exact formula when it comes to this aging process. No two people age exactly the same. There are many variables that will affect the long-term shape and health of your rear end. The NIH also says these variables and influences "include heredity, environment, culture, diet, exercise and leisure, past illnesses, and many other factors. ... Although some changes always occur with aging, they occur at different rates and to different extents. There is no way to predict exactly how you will age."[2]

However, there are still some things you can do to stay in the game as long as possible.

## Maintaining Your Shape

Just as your BBL is going to respond to aging and gravity the same as any other butt out there, it will also respond to proper nutrition and exercise. You can keep your derriere looking its best by staying committed to looking *your* best. Maintaining a healthy diet affects you from the inside out. Nutritional foods nourish your cells and keep them healthier longer. In addition, exercise will go a long way in keeping your butt looking its best as long as possible. Specifically, exercises that are targeted to that area. Keeping your glutes toned and strong will prevent some of the droop that comes with age.

In a study published in the Journal of Orthopedics and Sports Physical Therapy, researchers gathered data on 12 different exercises in order to identify which ones activated the glutes the most. They found the most effective exercises to be one-leg squats and one-leg deadlift exercises.[3] In addition to these exercises, celebrity personal trainer and fitness author Larysa DiDio suggests walking or running uphill, lunging, sprinting, and the glute bridge.[4]

Beyond diet and exercise, you can also look into additional cosmetic procedures to help you maintain your butt's shape. For example, a few decades after your fat transfer when there is a dramatic loss in your skin elasticity, resulting in a droopy hind end, we can actually surgically remove the skin at the top of the butt and lift the butt up again, just as suspenders are able to keep your pants from falling down.

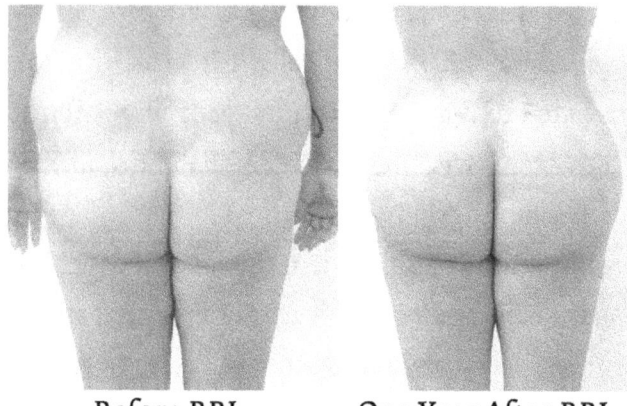

Before BBL      One Year After BBL

There are also non-surgical options to keep your butt lifted, such as skin tightening lasers. These treatments are good options to do every few years to maintain the skin firmness and elasticity and help fight the effects of gravity on your results.

## The Bottom Line

The bottom line is that the BBL doesn't prevent mother nature from doing her thing. Whatever you have is going to look droopier and saggier when you're older. This is true whether or not you have a BBL procedure. The question is, do you want to have a floppier, skinnier, deflated butt that looks saggy, or would you rather have a droopier, floppier butt that still has additional volume and shape to it? We are fortunate to have some pretty good tools and resources that allow us to stay in the game as long as possible and ward off gravity a little longer.

---

[1] "DIY Plastic Surgery Leads to Horrific Injuries," 2 July 2014; https://www.cnn.com/2014/07/01/health/diy-plastic-surgery/index.html.

[2] "Aging changes in organs, tissues, and cells;" 1, April 2019; https://medlineplus.gov/ency/article/004012.htm.

[3] "Gluteal muscle activation during common therapeutic exercises," Pubmed.org, 24 February 2009; https://www.ncbi.nlm.nih.gov/pubmed/19574661.

[4] Larysa DiDio, "My Butt Keeps Going South As I Age—Help," 29 April 2014; https://www.prevention.com/fitness/fitness-tips/a20457381/my-butt-keeps-going-south-as-i-age-help/.

# CHAPTER NINE
## *Team Work Makes the Dream Work*

As you make your decision to move forward with your Brazilian Butt Lift, my motto is simple: team work makes the dream work. Selecting the right team to handle your procedure is more than just comparing prices and bios. You want to find a team that you can trust and who will hold your hand and walk you through the entire process. That process begins well before you come in for surgery and extends far beyond. It comes down to customer service. How will you be treated before, during, and after your procedure?

## The Experience

As a surgeon, I don't operate in a vacuum. At Younique Surgery Center and Medical Spa, our team recognizes that we get one chance to make our first impression on you. We get one shot at wowing you with our skills, our history of results, and what you can expect from working with us. This is why we are extremely meticulous when it comes to creating a *total experience* for you. In our office, we have created an entire environment and culture around that experience.

Disneyland is a perfect example of what I'm talking about when it comes to creating an experience. If you've ever been, perhaps you've noticed that all the employees' name badges aren't just printouts of their names. Each name tag identifies each employee as a "cast member." From the person checking you into your hotel to the person responsible for removing the garbage, everyone is a cast member in the production that Disneyland is putting on for all of its customers. And it *is* a production! Being "the happiest place on Earth" is not just about the rides and having fun—it's about an experience. It's about a *feeling*. The difference between

Disneyland and all other amusement parks is how you *feel* when you leave. It's guaranteed.

That's on purpose.

Just like Disneyland, our practice in Santa Monica, California, works to create a specific experience for you. When you walk into our office, you are greeted warmly by a friendly face. You might notice the pleasant smell of our aroma therapy and candles. You will enjoy the gourmet refreshments we stock in the waiting area. When it's time for your procedure, you will be wrapped in a warm, fluffy robe instead of a paper gown. All of this is targeted to make you feel a certain way—like you are a part of our family. The culture here is designed so that you don't feel as if you're walking into a cold, sterile, medical office—you feel as if you're coming *home*.

All of this is so important because at the end of the day, you're not going to go home and talk with your family members and friends about the actual procedure or detail the instruments we used in the process and exactly how many cc's of fat were transferred. When you're sitting down and talking about your experience with us, you're going to be talking about what it was like for you, which is specifically shaped by your feelings about your experiences with us. You are going to talk to them about how you felt before, during, and after the procedure because that is what will stay with you.

## Staying in Touch

All of these touch points before, during, and after your procedure are extremely important to us. When somebody comes to a consultation, we follow up by sending a thank you card. It's just a note to say, "Thank you for coming and trusting us to handle your cosmetic goals—we look forward to you having the procedure with us. By the way, here's more information about what we discussed." We send our patients this information even if they choose to have their procedure somewhere else because we want you to have all the information to make the right decision. We believe that educated patients make the best decisions for themselves. We stay in constant communication with you, even after the procedure is done.

This is especially true for the time during your

recovery period. We talked in earlier chapters about that happiness curve. That happiness curve shows how you're going to be feeling during the life of your BBL experience, and right after the procedure, you're going to be in a very vulnerable place. You will be sore, you will be bruised, and you may be wondering why you agreed to undergo the procedure at all. This can be an ugly phase for some of our patients. It's scary. We make a point to walk that road with you and very literally hold your hand through that part of your journey. We go out of our way to soften this difficult period of time for you and give you the emotional and physical support you need for a smooth transition into the peak of that happiness curve where you are excited and joyful about your procedure.

Beyond your recovery period, we are still there checking in with you to see how things are going. We try to maintain an open dialogue with you at all times. After your procedure, we see you at one week, one month, six weeks, six months, twelve months, and beyond. We make sure that not only are you healing right, but that you're also happy with your results. Once you've moved into the top of that happiness curve, we still want to support you as you move forward. On your one-year anniversary, we send a "birthday" card just to let you know we're still thinking of you and care, and that we're happy to help you with any of your future cosmetic needs. We aim to keep a consistent pulse on your emotional well-being just as you would expect any other family member to do.

This idea of belonging is a very intentional part of what we try to create for you, both when you come in, when you leave, and at every point in between. The way we create this culture is both a personal and business practice.

Starbucks is great example of this. You or someone you know is probably a raving fan of Starbucks. But why do you pay two to three times more for coffee at Starbucks rather than just making a quick stop at the BP gas station or going through the drive-thru at McDonald's for coffee? The reason is that you aren't paying extra for coffee at all. You're paying for the *experience*. If you blind taste McDonald's versus Starbucks brews, people aren't necessarily going to say the cheaper one is terrible, and they may not even notice much of a difference at all. However, if you compare the two experiences, there is a night and day difference.

When you walk through the doors of a Starbucks you've been to before, the barista is likely to know your name. He or she will look at you with a familiar smile and ask if you want the usual—the way you always like it. They know what kind of milk you prefer, how much sugar you want, and exactly how you're going to order it. Two minutes later, you're leaving with a smile on your face before you've even had your first sip. People pay more for coffee at their local Starbucks for the same reason people pay over $100 to spend a day at Disneyland when they could have gone to a carnival down the road for a quarter of the price to spend the day on rides. People *want* the experience of feeling welcome and happy.

That's exactly what we are trying to do for you—the patient. When you leave our practice, I want you to feel better about yourself inside and out. I want you to have more confidence, to be happy, and to feel satisfied when you look in the mirror and see you have achieved the cosmetic goals you wanted to achieve when you walked into my practice. We understand that those kinds of results are just about precision in the surgical room. We achieve them with intention every step of the way before, during, and after the procedure itself.

## I Promise to Put You...Second!

One of the ways I work to create this experience for you is by promising to always put you second. You're probably thinking, *What do you mean*, second?! I agree, it does sound counterintuitive. However, let me explain.

As the boss and the surgeon, I put my patients second and my *employees* first. The reason I do this is because I know that if I treat my employees well and like family, they are going to emulate that and pass that same treatment on to you. So, in putting my employees first, I ensure that my patients come first for everyone else. Just like all staff members at Disneyland are considered cast members in the performance that is the experience of Disneyland, so are each of my staff members a touch point in your experience with me.

This is why I work so hard to create the feel of

family within my office. There are many things we do together as boss and employees. We always make sure we work together as a team. We do fun things together such as going bowling or having ice skating nights. Each year, we do a team retreat at a fun destination. I rent a huge estate for four or five days, and we just stay in. This allows us to get to know each other on the tennis courts, over the grill, hiking on the trails, sitting together in a painting class, or sipping wine after dinner. We spend the entirety of the trip bonding as family. The more we know about each other on that kind of personal level, the more we are able to work together as a team. And remember, team work makes the dream work. By that, I mean *your* dream. You have a beautiful vision of what you want, and it's our job to work together to make that dream come true.

It's so important to me that my staff and I have this kind of relationship because I know patients can sense that. When you come for a consult, you can sense whether staff members like each other or not. If you know they do, you will also know you are going to have a good experience with us. You know that the team is working together to take care of you. You can sense whether or not we're working together to make that happen. That culture starts with me—the boss—and trickles down into every detail of our office. I treat my staff like family in order to guarantee that you will then have a perfect experience with *all* of us.

Often, patients are scared and nervous the day of their surgeries. When I walk through the door to mark their bodies before we begin, the first thing they ask me is, "Doctor, did you get a good night's sleep? How's your mood today? Are you feeling happy?" They aren't just making friendly conversation. They are looking for reassurance that I'm ready—mentally, physically, and emotionally.

And so I grin and tell them the truth. "I am feeling wonderful. I love my job, and we're going to have a great day together." It puts a huge smile on their faces, and it puts them at ease. That's what they want to feel—that confidence that we really are going to have a good day together, and that they are literally in safe hands. They want to know that everyone is ready, in a good mood, and excited to have them there.

Unhappy employees don't last very long in our practice. If employees ever walk into my office with a sour look on their faces—maybe they woke up on the wrong side of the bed or they are dealing with a difficult personal matter—they have to leave their issues at the door or I send them home because they have to be happy on the inside in order to make other people happy on their insides. It's infectious. And inside my surgery room, it's Disneyland—regardless of what is going on in their personal lives.

It has to be this way because your experience as the patient is the most important thing to me. It also makes it a happier work environment for everyone.

## Our Specialty

One of the reasons we are so confident in our ability to provide you with such a powerful and safe experience is that the Brazilian Butt Lift is one of just a few things we offer in our office. We invest our efforts and our study into a small number of procedures and services in order to give you the best experience possible. You aren't going to come in to our office and see four hundred different services on the menu. I feel strongly about not diluting my expertise. (Think of the old adage *Jack of all trades, master of none*.) You are most likely to have a great experience when the whole team, including the surgeon, focuses only on a few procedures they do well. I can do everything—but I'm the best at the few things I have mastered. When you come to our office for the BBL procedure, you can be sure that my team and I are going to be laser focused on making it the best procedure possible *because* we don't do everything. We just do a few things very well.

Now you have a better idea of who we are. But you don't have to take our word for it. You will see that the many, many reviews of our office on Google and Yelp give evidence that we deliver on our first impression. By the time you come into our office, we know that you have likely Googled or Yelped us and read the reviews to see what other people are saying about us. We know that we can't fake our way through that first impression, *especially* when we are working with educated patients like yourself. We understand that it's important to you to see how we handle unhappy and dissatisfied patients, how we respond to negative reviews, and how we take care of patients who have had to make an adjustment to their surgeries. We understand that you are looking for those kinds of examples in order to get an idea of how we address concerns with patients before and after surgery. We encourage you to do your research because we are extremely confident that the data stacks in our favor. As a general rule, we strive to under-promise and over-deliver.

As you do your research in order to determine whether the BBL is right for you and then choose the practitioner who will serve you best, we hope that you'll come to the same conclusion we have—that we can't *wait* for you to come join our family!

# Conclusion

I hope this book has been a helpful conversation for you. It has been my intention to give you all the information you need in order to choose—for yourself—if the Brazilian Butt Lift is right for you. As you can see, there are several factors to consider when making this decision. It should not be taken lightly, but you *can* make it wisely.

I encourage you to always ask the right questions from the right people. There will always be those who want to put in their two cents on your decisions for a variety of reasons. I hope this book will assist you in cutting through the noise so that you can tap in to your own sense of desire and vision. What do *you* want? How do you want to celebrate your own beauty? How do you want to experience your body?

I have done—and will continue to do—my best in assisting you throughout that decision-making process, but these are intimate questions that you alone will need to answer.

As both a cosmetic surgeon and an artist, I love the role I get to play in helping women shape themselves and their lives into all they imagined it could become. I firmly believe that this power to choose should be in your hands, and that you should guard that power fiercely. Never make this decision because someone else wants you to. On the flip side of that, don't let others sway you from taking this step if your heart is set on taking it.

Follow where your heart leads you. And if it happens to lead you to my office—the happiest place on earth for cosmetic surgery—I will welcome you with open arms. I'm in the business of making dreams come true, and I will always do my best to make yours come true for you. In the meantime, your job is to dream them. So, keep dreaming and trust that there's a path to get you there.

Don't worry. Your heart will know the way home—wherever that happens to be for *you*.

# Appendix

# The Brazilian Butt Lift FAQs

### What is a Brazilian Butt Lift?

The Brazilian Butt Lift is a procedure in which the surgeon takes excess fat from other areas of your body such as your thighs, flanks, or abdomen, and then deposits it into your butt to make it fuller and more lifted.

### What's the difference between the BBL and implants?

The BBL uses your own fat, whereas an implant uses artificial silicone implants. The BBL is much safer and more natural looking because you are using your body's own resources. Implants pose an increased risk of infection and other complications.

## What types of results can I expect from the BBL?

We strategically add the additional fat to your butt in the spots where it will give the most desired effect. The BBL will naturally lift and round your bottom to give it a smoother and more attractive look.

## What can I expect during the BBL consultation?

This will be an opportunity for you to ask all of your questions and discuss your specific goals with your surgeon. During this time, the doctor will able to determine whether you are a good candidate for the procedure, or whether you should consider alternatives. We will talk to you about the BBL procedure itself, including the associated risks and benefits. The goal of the consultation is to give you all the information you need in order to make an educated and informed decision about whether or not the BBL is right for you. The consultation also allows the surgeon to determine what buttocks shape you are looking for.

## Who is a Good Candidate for the BBL?

The ideal candidate for the BBL is normal weight or even slightly overweight in order to ensure that there is enough fat on the body that can be transferred to the butt. Patients who are too thin will not have enough fat for the transfer, and patients who are over a body mass index of thirty-two are at a higher risk for complications with anesthesia. However, patients in either the too-thin or too-heavy category can consider either gaining or losing weight for the purpose of this surgery. This will be discussed during your consultation.

## Can I get the BBL if I'm thin?

The ideal candidate for the BBL is normal weight or even slightly overweight in order to ensure that there is enough fat on the body that can be transferred to the butt. However, if you do not currently have enough fat, we can discuss the possibility of you gaining some weight for the purpose of the procedure. The surgeon can also discuss butt implants as a last resort.

## What does a BBL procedure entail?

During the procedure, your surgeon uses liposuction to gather excess fat from your thighs, flanks, and/or abdomen. The fat is then purified before being injected into your buttocks. The injections are done in a strategic way to give your butt the best aesthetic outcome in terms of lift, shape, and projection.

## How safe is the BBL procedure?

The BBL is the safest way to cosmetically alter the shape of your butt because you are using your own fat to do so, as opposed to introducing foreign materials into the body to get the look you want. However, there are still some risks involved because it is an invasive surgery that requires anesthesia. There is a small risk for infection, hematoma, seroma formation, and even death, but these risks are greatly reduced as you follow the thorough post-op instructions provided.

## How long before I can sit after the BBL procedure?

Try to completely avoid sitting or laying on the fat graft site for the first three weeks after the surgery, and only when necessary through the fourth week. When you have to sit, use a Boppy pillow to help reduce the pressure on the site. Placing too much pressure on the graft can cause you to lose volume because the cells will die more rapidly.

## How long will it take to recover after the BBL is performed?

Recovery time is about four weeks, with most patients being cleared to go back to work the third week after surgery. You should definitely expect to be out of work for the first two weeks, and you will be required to have someone with you for the first twenty-four hours. Ideally, you will have a caretaker with you for the first week, as you will likely be taking prescription pain medications and unable to drive.

## How long does it take to see the permanent results of the BBL?

Your butt will go through a few phases following the BBL procedure before finally stabilizing in size and shape at around three to six months. In the first two weeks after the graft, your butt will lose up to 40 percent of its initial volume. This is normal, and we overfill in the first place to compensate for this. After that, the stem cells in your butt begin to regenerate and produce additional fat cells, which will cause an increase in volume. Finally, everything stabilizes between three and six months.

## How long does the BBL last?

Your BBL can last for decades! You can expect to retain 50 to 60 percent of the initial fat transfer for the lifetime of your BBL. This is a semi-permanent procedure simply because the nature of your fat is only semi-permanent. Your butt will change over time as it responds to the normal aging process, whether or not you gain or lose substantial amounts of weight, and your overall diet. For best results, maintain an active and healthy lifestyle without extreme changes in your weight.

## Will the BBL require additional procedures over the years?

The BBL will potentially last for decades without the need for additional procedures. However, some patients opt to come in during their later years for a lift procedure to combat sagging due to the normal aging process. Others may choose to do occasional skin tightening procedures to maintain their results.

## If I'm not a good candidate for the BBL, what are my alternatives?

If for any reason you are not deemed a good fit for the BBL, you can consider getting silicone implants or filler injections. However, the BBL will give the best and most long-term results, so this should be the first choice for any patient who qualifies.

## How much does a BBL cost?

The cost will vary depending on how much work needs to be done in order to achieve your specific goals. This will be determined by variables such as your body type, how much fat you want transferred, and the current shape and volume of your back-end. In order to get the most accurate pricing for your specific procedure and find out about our different pricing options, it's best to contact our office and schedule an in-person consultation.

# Preparing For Your Surgery: At a Glance

It's important to be thorough in your preparation beforehand keeping in mind that our instructions are meant to ensure your overall safety, a smooth procedure, and a fast recovery period.

## Four Weeks Prior to Surgery

- Stop the use of all nicotine products. There is to be absolutely no smoking or nicotine use for the month before and after your surgery. Zero! This is because nicotine use can reduce your blood flow, which results in an overall decrease in the oxygenation of your blood and body. Specifically, this means that the cut edges of your incisions are not going to have the oxygen and nutrients they need to heal properly. Poor healing can lead to undesirable scars or even skin breakdown during recovery.

## Two Weeks Prior to Surgery

- No aspirin or medicines that contain aspirin* because it interferes with normal blood clotting.
- No ibuprofen or medicines that contain ibuprofen* because it interferes with blood clotting.
- Discontinue all herbal medications* because many have side effects that could complicate a surgical procedure by inhibiting blood clotting, affecting blood pressure, or interfering with anesthetics.
- Discontinue all diet pills—whether prescription, over-the-counter, or herbal—as many will interfere with anesthesia and can cause cardiovascular concerns.

- No megadoses of Vitamin E, although a multiple vitamin that contains Vitamin E is fine to take up to one week prior and you can resume one week after surgery.
- Absolutely no smoking because nicotine reduces blood flow to the skin and can cause significant complications during healing.
- Start taking the recommended supplements each day and continue taking this through your recovery. The healthier you are, the quicker your recovery will be.

* See *Medications to Avoid* in the Appendix

## One Week Prior to Surgery

- Do not take or drink any alcohol or drugs beginning one week prior to your surgery and until at least one week after your surgery, as these can interfere with anesthesia and affect blood clotting.
- Do not take any cough or cold medications without permission.

- Begin using a germ-inhibiting soap for bathing, such as Dial, Safeguard, or Lever (as long as your skin can tolerate it).
- Report any signs of cold, infection, boils, or pustules appearing before surgery.
- Make arrangements for a responsible adult to drive you to and from the facility on the day of your surgery. You will not be allowed to leave on your own.
- Make arrangements for a responsible individual to spend the first twenty-four hours with you. You cannot be left alone.

## Night Prior to and Morning of Surgery

- Do not eat or drink anything (not even water) after midnight the night before your surgery and until after the surgery. Do not sneak anything, as this may endanger you.
- Clear any regular medications you're taking with your surgeon beforehand.
- Take a thorough shower with germ-inhibiting soap the night before and the morning of surgery.

## PREPARING FOR YOUR SURGERY: AT A GLANCE

- Be sure to shampoo or shave your underarm and pubic hair the morning of surgery. This is to decrease the bacteria on the skin, which will thereby decrease the risk of infection.
- Do not apply any of the following to your skin, hair, or face the morning of surgery: makeup, cream, lotion, hair gel, body spray, perfume, powder, or deodorant. Using any of these products will add bacteria to the skin and increase the risk of infection.
- You may brush your teeth the morning of surgery, but do not drink anything.
- Do not wear contacts to surgery. If you bring glasses, bring your eyeglass case.
- Wear comfortable, loose-fitting clothes that do not have to be put on over your head. The best thing to wear home is a button-up top and pull-on pants. You will also want flat shoes that are easy to slip on.
- Do not bring any valuables or wear any jewelry (no rings, earrings, chains, toe rings, other metal piercings, or watches). We will need to tape wedding rings if worn.

- You must have another adult drive you to and from surgery. Please note that a cab or bus driver will not be allowed to take you home after surgery. On arrival, be sure we know your drivers' names, phone numbers, and how we will be able to reach them.

# Pre-Operative Shopping List

Following is a list of items that should be purchased prior to surgery in order to prepare and recover from surgery.

| Have | Need | |
|---|---|---|
| | | **Prescriptions** – please have your prescriptions filled prior to surgery |
| | | **Tylenol** (or a generic form of this drug) – this will be the drug of choice once you do not need the prescription-strength pain medications |
| | | **Arnica Montana** – to take prior to surgery and during your recovery. You can purchase these products at GNC or Vitamin Shoppe or Whole Foods Market |

| HAVE | NEED | |
|---|---|---|
| | | **Germ-inhibiting soap,** such as Dial, Safeguard, or Lever 2000 – to bathe with prior to surgery in order to minimize germs. |
| | | **Personal Grooming** – such as shaving the surgical area, removing nail polish (light color), and tying your hair back. |
| | | **Straws** – you need to drink lots of fluids after surgery in order to help get the anesthesia out of your body quicker, and straws helps you drink more. |
| | | **Boppy Pillow** – necessary for fat transfer to buttocks. You can find this at any store in the baby aisle (must bring the day of surgery). |

## Gentle Foods – to encourage eating and not upset the stomach initially:

| HAVE | NEED | |
|---|---|---|
| | | **Gatorade** (for at least the next 2-5 days after surgery) |
| | | **Toast, plain crackers, saltines (not buttery)** |
| | | **Soups** (water-based, not cream-based) |
| | | **Puddings, applesauce, Jello** |

PRE-OPERATIVE SHOPPING LIST

| **AVOID:** | |
|---|---|
| | **Salt** – this will cause swelling. |
| | **Dairy Products** – this will cause nausea |
| | **Attire** – please wear loose fitting clothing with opening in the front and remove all piercings and jewelry. |
| | **Surgery Confirmation** – your surgery arrival time should be confirmed the day before; be available for instructions. |

# Post-Operative Instructions

The following instructions should be followed closely except when overruled by specific procedural instructions. You must follow your surgeon's instructions as indicated for your specific surgery. Notify the doctor of any changes in your condition and call the office with any questions.

- You MUST HAVE AN ADULT DRIVE YOU HOME from the facility. You will not be allowed to drive yourself or use public transportation.
- After surgery you MUST HAVE A RESPONSIBLE ADULT STAY WITH YOU a minimum

of twenty-four hours. You CANNOT be left alone. The twenty-four hours begin when you are discharged from the office or hospital. Have everything ready at home PRIOR to surgery. Make arrangements for someone to stay with you. Let the person or persons know you cannot be left alone. This is important because of the danger of falling and you may lose the concept of time for the day and overmedicate yourself.

- The effects of anesthesia can persist for twenty-four hours. You must exercise extreme caution before engaging in any activity that could be harmful to yourself or others.
- DRINK fluids to help rid the body of the drugs used in surgery. If you have straws in the house, you will tend to drink more fluids the first few days after surgery.
- Resume your normal diet as tolerated. Eating foods that are bland and soft, however, may be best tolerated during the first day or so. You must eat more than crackers and juice, otherwise you will continue to feel weak and will not heal as well.

- REMEMBER to take the medications with a little something to eat or you may experience increased nausea.
- Please avoid the use of alcoholic beverages for the first seven days (it dilates blood vessels and can cause unwanted bleeding) and as long as pain medications are being used (dangerous combination).
- Take only medications that have been prescribed by your surgeon for your postoperative care and take them according to the instruction on the bottle. Your pain medication may make you feel "spacey"; therefore, have someone else give you your medications according to the proper time intervals.
- If you experience any generalized itching, rash, wheezing or tightness in the throat, stop taking all medications and call the office immediately, as this may be a sign of a drug allergy.
- You can expect moderate discomfort, which should be helped by the pain medications. The greatest discomfort is usually during the

first forty-eight hours. Thereafter, you will find that you require less pain medication.

- Call your doctor's office if you have: SEVERE PAIN that is not responding to pain medication; swelling that is greater on one side than the other; incisions that are RED OR FEVERISH; a FEVER; or if any other questions or problems arise.
- Keep any DRESSINGS ON, CLEAN, AND DRY. Do not remove them until instructed to do so. There may be some bloody drainage on the dressings. If you have excessive bleeding or the bandages are too tight, call the office immediately.
- After surgery it is important to have a bowel movement within a day or two. If you do not, you may take over the counter laxatives to encourage your bowels to move.
- Minimal activity for the first forty-eight hours. No house cleaning, furniture rearranging, etc. Relax, be pampered, and let your body heal. The less energy you use on doing things, the more energy your body can focus on healing.

- Limit lifting, pulling or pushing for fourteen days. No lifting over five pounds for the first two weeks.
- You are requested to remain within a reasonable traveling distance of your doctor's office for approximately seven days.
- Once cleared to shower, you may do so every day. Please do not use the bathtub for two weeks.
- NO SMOKING for the first fourteen postoperative days. Any cheating will delay healing and may lead to severe complications.
- You may drive two days after anesthesia, once you are off the pain pills, and when you experience no pain with this activity (you need to be able to react quickly).
- All surgeries involve some scarring, which can take up to a year to fade. No matter how small they may be, we still want them to heal as well as they are able. Exposing red scars to the sun can cause permanent discoloration. A good sunscreen (SPF 30 or higher) can help and will protect the surrounding tissues that might not feel a sunburn developing while

the nerves are healing. Sunlight can even reach scars under a swimsuit, so take adequate precautions.

- DO NOT use a hot tub for four weeks.
- AVOID sports or strenuous activities four to six weeks as your surgeon gives you clearance during your postoperative visits. This is to avoid any unnecessary complications (bleeding, bruising, swelling).
- You may return to work when you feel able and are cleared to do so by your surgeon.

# Medications to Avoid

If you are taking any medications on this list, they should be discontinued two weeks prior to surgery. Only acetaminophen products, such as Tylenol, should be taken for pain.

Avoid *all* diet aids, including over-the-counter and herbal products, as these intensify anesthesia, which can cause serious cardiovascular effects.

All other medications—prescriptions, over-the-counter, and herbal—that you are currently taking must be specifically cleared by your surgeon prior to surgery.

# Aspirin-like Medications to Avoid
*The following medications can affect blood clotting*

4-Way Cold Tabs
5-Aminosalicylic Acid
　Acetilsalicylic Acid
Actron
Adprin-B products
Aleve
Alka-Seltzer products
　Amigesic Argesic-SA
　Anacin products
Anexsia w/Codeine Arthra-G
Arthriten products Arthritis
　Foundation products
Arthritis Pain Formula
Arthritis Strength BC
Powder
Arthropan
ASA
Asacol
Ascriptin products Aspergum
　Asprimox products
Axotal Azdone
Azulfidine products
B-A-C
Backache Maximum Strength
　Relief Bayer Products
BC Powder
Bismatrol products Buffered
　Aspirin
Bufferin products

Buffetts 11
Buffex
Butal/ASA/Caff
Butalbital Compound Cama
　Arthritis Pain Reliever
Carisoprodol Compound
Cataflam
Cheracol
Choline Magnesium
Trisalicylate
Choline Salicylate
Cope Coricidin
Cortisone Medications
Damason-P
Darvon Compound-65
Darvon/ASA
Diclofenac
Dipentum
Disalcid
Doan's products
Dolobid
Dristan
Duragesic
Easprin
Ecotrin products Empirin
　products Equagesic
Etodolac
Excedrin products
Fiorgen PF

Fiorinal products
Flurbiprofen
Gelpirin
Genprin
Gensan
Goody's Extra Strength
  Headache Powders
  Halfprin products
IBU
Indomethacin products
Isollyl Improved
Kaodene
Lanorinal
Ibuprohm
Lodine
Lortab ASA
Magan
Magnaprin products
Magnesium Salicylate
Magsal
Marnal
Marthritic
Mefenamic Acid
Meprobamate
Mesalamine
Methocarbamol
Micrainin
Mobidin
Mobigesic
Momentum
Mono-Gesic
Motrin products

Naprelan
Naproxen
Night-Time Effervescent Cold
Norgesic products Norwich
  products Olsalazine
Orphengesic products Orudis
  products Oxycodone
  Pabalate products
P-A-C
Pain Reliever Tabs Panasal
  Pentasa
Pepto-Bismol
Percodan products
Phenaphen/Codeine #3
Pink Bismuth
Piroxicam
Propoxyphene
Compound products
Robaxisal
Rowasa
Roxeprin
Saleto products
Salflex
Salicylate products
Salsalate
Salsitab
Scot-Tussin Original 5-
  Action
Sine-off
Sinutab
Sodium Salicylate
Sodol Compound

MEDICATIONS TO AVOID

Soma Compound
St. Joseph Aspirin
Sulfasalazine
Supac
Suprax
Synalgos-DC
Talwin
Triaminicin
Tricosal

Trilisate
Tussanil DH
Tussirex products
Ursinus-lnlay
Vanquish
Wesprin
Willow Bark products
Zorprin

## Ibuprofen-like Medications to Avoid

Acular
 (opthalmic)
Advil products
Anaprox
 products
Ansaid
Clinoril
Daypro
Dimetapp Sinus
Dristan Sinus
Feldene
Fenoprofen
Genpril
Haltran
Ibuprin
Ibuprofen
Indochron E-R

Indocin
 products
Ketoprofen
Ketorolac
Meclofenamate
Meclomen
Menadol
Midol-products
Nabumetone
Nalfon
 products
Naprosyn
 products
Naprox
Nuprin
Ocufen
 (opthalmic)

Oruvail
Oxaprozin
Ponstel
Profenal
Relafen
Rhinocaps
Sine-Aid
 products
Sulindac
Suprofen
Tolectin
 products
Tolmetin
Toradol
Voltaren

## Antidepressant Medications to Avoid

*The following medications can intensify anesthesia and have cardiovascular effects*

| | |
|---|---|
| Ad a pin | Limbitrol products |
| Amitriptyline | Ludiomil |
| Amoxapine | Maprotiline |
| Anafranil | Norpramin |
| Asendin | Nortriptyline |
| Aventyl | Pamelor |
| Clomipramine | Pertofrane |
| Desipramine | Protriptyline |
| Doxepin | Sinequan |
| Elavil | Surmontil |
| Endep | Tofranil |
| Etrafon products | Triavil |
| Imipramine | Trimipramine |
| Janimine | Vivactil |

## Other Medications to Avoid

*The following medications can affect blood clotting*

| | | |
|---|---|---|
| 4-Way w/ Codeine A.C.A. | Anturane | Coumadin |
| A-A Compound | Arthritis | Dalteparin injection |
| Accutrim | Bufferin | Dicumerol |
| Actifed | BC Tablets | Dipyridamole |
| Anexsia | Childrens Advil | Doxycycline |
| Anisindione | Clinoril | Emagrin |
| | Contac | |

MEDICATIONS TO AVOID

| | | |
|---|---|---|
| Enoxaparin injection | Miradon | Sparine |
| Flagyl | Opasal | Stelazine |
| Fragmin injection | Pan-PAC | Sulfinpyrazone |
| Furadantin | Pentoxyfylline | Tenuate |
| Garlic | Persantine | Tenuate Dospan |
| Heparin | Phenylpropanolamine | Thorazine |
| Hydrocortisone | Prednisone | Ticlid |
| Isollyl | Protamine | Ticlopidine |
| Lovenox injection | Pyrroxate | Trental |
| Macrodantin | Ru-Tuss | Ursinus |
| Mellaril | Salatin | Virbamycin |
| | Sinex | Vitamin E |
| | Sofarin | Warfarin |
| | Soltice | |

## Salicylate Medications, Foods & Beverages to Avoid

*The following foots and medications can affect blood clotting*

- Almonds
- Amigesic (salsalate)
- Apples
- Apricots
- Blackberries
- Boysenberries
- Cherries
- Chinese black beans
- Cucumbers
- Currants
- Disalcid (salsalate)
- Doan's (magnesium salicylate)
- Dolobid (diflunisal)
- Garlic
- Ginger
- Grapes
- Magsal

Mobigesic
Pabalate
Pamprin (Max. Pain Relief)
Pickles
Prunes
Pepto-Bismol (bismuth subsalicylate)
Raspberries
Salflex (salsalate)
Salsalate
Salsitab (salsalate)
Strawberries
Tomatoes
Trilisate (choline salicylate + magnesium salicylate
Wine

## Vitamins and Herbs to Avoid

*The following vitamins and herbs can affect blood clotting, blood sugar, increase or decrease the strength of anesthesia, cause rapid heartbeat, cause high blood pressure, and liver damage.* **Note:** *If your vitamin or herb is not listed here, please do not assume that it is safe to take while preparing your for your BBL.*

Ackee fruit
Alfalfa
Aloe
Argimony
Barley
Bilberry
Bitter melon
Burdock root
Carrot oil
Cayenne
Chamomile
Chromium
Coriander
Dandelion root
Devil's club
Dong Quai root
Echinacea
Ephedra
Eucalyptus
Fenugreek seeds
Feverfew
Fo-ti
Garlic
Ginger
Gingko
Gingo biloba
Ginseng
Gmena
Goldenseal
Gotu Kola
Guarana
Guayusa
Hawthorn
Horse Chestnut

## MEDICATIONS TO AVOID

- Juniper
- Kava Kava
- Lavender
- Lemon verbena
- Licorice root
- Ma Huang
- Melatonin
- Muwort
- Nem seed oil
- Onions
- Papaya
- Periwinkle
- Selenium
- St. John's Wort
- Valerian root
- The Natural Viagra®
- Vitamin E
- Willow bark
- Yellow root
- Yohim

www.ingramcontent.com/pod-product-compliance
Lightning Source LLC
Chambersburg PA
CBHW051359290426
44108CB00015B/2075